# IT'S ALL IN YOUR HEAD

## The Link Between Mercury Amalgams and Illness

# DR. HAL A. HUGGINS

 AVERY PUBLISHING GROUP INC.

Garden City Park, New York

Cover designers: Rudy Shur and Ann Vestal
Cover computer graphics © Digital Art/Westlight
In-house editor: Amy C. Tecklenburg
Typesetter: Bonnie Freid
Printer: Paragon Press, Honesdale, PA


The excerpts on pages 43–44 and 47–48 are reprinted with the
permission of Dr. Douglas Swartzendruber.

**Library of Congress Cataloging-in-Publication Data**

Huggins, Hal A.
    It's all in your head : the link between mercury amalgams and
illness / Hal A. Huggins
      p. cm.
    Includes bibliographical references and index.
    ISBN 0-89529-550-4
    1. Mercury—Toxicology. 2. Dental amalgams—Toxicology.
I. Title.
RA1231.M5H84 1993          93-4660
615.9'25663—dc20          CIP

Printed in the United States of America.

10  9  8

# Contents

# Foreword

Dr. Hal Huggins has spearheaded what will go down in medical history as one of the most remarkable movements of rebellion against medical—or in this case dental—tyranny and obstinate pigheadedness ever recorded. And some day, when that rebellion has attained complete success—and it will—we all ought to thank him for it.

Certainly it's fair to say that if Hal Huggins hadn't been banging the drums to alert us to the dangers of the mercury in our dental fillings, it would have taken many more years before public awareness rose to even the level it has currently reached. Hal wasn't afraid to take on the American Dental Association over silver-mercury amalgams, and in recent years he's been equally willing to expose the dangers of root canals.

All of this has made a significant difference in my medical practice, and it's made me aware of the importance of cooperation and teamwork between doctors and dentists. The simple and overwhelmingly significant truth is this: *What happens to your teeth can affect your entire body.*

When patients tell me, "Doctor, for the past two years I've been suffering from overwhelming fatigue. I don't have the slightest idea what happened to me," one of the first questions I ask is, "Did you have any dental work done around the time you first began feeling so tired?" A very large percentage of the time, the answer is yes.

Is this a coincidence? I used to ask myself. It was no coincidence. Soon I began asking other categories of patients the same question. Not just chronic-fatiguers, but people with yeast infections, multiple sclerosis, and other neurological disorders often said yes. I was finding out that Dr. Hal Huggins was on to something.

I don't suppose I have to tell you that mercury is a deadly poison and that it doesn't belong in our mouths. Hal is going to explain that in detail. What I've learned in working with patients is that many people who have silver-mercury amalgams and many people who have root-canal work have simply stepped over the boundary between what their immune systems can tolerate and what they can't. When they do that the message their bodies send is frequently a frightening one.

Dentists are going to have to accept responsibility for the medical problems their techniques create. More importantly, they're going to have to listen to Dr. Huggins and stop delivering dangerous treatments to their unsuspecting patients. I'm quite conscious of the fact that most dentists are men and women of good will who don't know any better. That situation, however, is going to change, and I hope that as it does, more and more conscientious dental professionals are going to join the rebellion against their own organization, the American Dental Association.

We physicians can't afford to be smug. We have our own problems with treatments whose high risk frequently diminishes the intended health benefit toward the vanishing point. (Take a look at the real statistics for heart bypass surgery, and you'll know just what I mean.)

What's essential is that all of us should look to those medical pioneers who are courageous enough to charge full tilt at the fortified ramparts of conventional medical care. The people I'm speaking of do not oppose the status quo out of any misguided hunger for controversy and notoriety; they do it because compelling medical evidence has shown them that concealed within "standard operating procedures" are real and preventable dangers for the folks who really matter in medicine—our patients.

Hal Huggins is one of the most distinguished of these pioneers. He is offering dentistry a chance to reform itself and be the important healing art that it can be. Someday we will see the changes he is heralding come to pass, and we will be the better for it.

Robert C. Atkins, M.D.

# Preface

*I*t's *All in Your Head* was written in response to the thousands of calls I have received from frustrated people who had just learned that their fillings contained mercury. Some people wanted the fillings removed immediately, and they wanted to know whom they should see, because their dentists had just told them that they were crazy. "Mercury is the safest and longest-lasting common filling that dentistry has to offer," would be the retort. The worst calls, however, came from those who had just had their fillings removed, and who now reported that they were in worse shape than they had ever been. I was frustrated too, because I knew that mercury is toxic, yet the leaders of organized dentistry insisted, "It is safe because we have used it for over 100 years."

This is the third time that the mercury debate has arisen. In the 1840s, according to dental lore, European dentists who used the new, cheap, poisonous mercury (quaksilber) fillings were called quaks. Translated into English, quaksilber was called quicksilver, and quak became quack. That era of dentistry is affectionately called Amalgam War One. Amalgam is the generic term for the most commonly used dental filling in the world, silver-mercury amalgam. This pastelike material is a combination of powdered compounds of copper, tin, silver, and zinc, which are added to equal amounts of liquid mercury and mixed together. The combination is then implanted in teeth.

Amalgam War One in the United States resulted in the 1840 demise of the National Association of Dental Surgeons. This association would ban as unethical any dentist who used mercury in a patient. When half the dentists used it anyway, the effectiveness of the organization was lost and it disintegrated into oblivion. Later, it was to be replaced by the American Dental Association (ADA), which favored the use of cheaper mercury fillings over more costly, but safer, gold fillings.

Amalgam War Two came along in the 1920s, led by Alfred Stock, Ph.D. Dr. Stock was a German chemist who himself became forgetful, brainfogged, and ill due to exposure to mercury from his fillings. Upon the removal of his fillings, he noted the return of his intellectual capacities, and he thought it only proper to warn his scientific colleagues of the toxicity of mercury from fillings. He published about thirty scientific articles on the subject, which met with interest from his peers, but with violent reactions from the dental community. After tolerating an inordinate amount of abuse from the dental organizations, he finally dropped the subject, and dentistry continued to place amalgam.

Amalgam War Three started in Mexico City, when Olympio Pinto, C.D., and I had an argument about the safety of dental amalgam. I argued for two hours that mercury did not come out of fillings, and that if it were a hazard, the ADA, the AMA, the FDA, the CIA, the FBI, and all the three-initialed agencies I could think of would certainly protect us. After all, that was what they were there for. Well, that was the old Huggins. I barely remember him now. The new Huggins emerged as the old one shut up and began to listen.

Dr. Pinto began to describe events of the 1920s. During that time, his dentist father removed amalgam and saw patients suffering from leukemia and neurological diseases improve. His father got the idea from an old journal. Dr. Pinto also described events of the early 1960s, when he himself came to America to earn a post-doctoral master's degree at Georgetown University. His chemistry and physics professors were very supportive about his thesis subject: the diseases caused by silver-mercury fillings. However, after he spent over one year struggling in his endeavor to prove mercury toxicity, the National Institute of Dental Research (NIDR)—just a few miles away—got wind of his research. Words were exchanged between the Georgetown professors and NIDR researchers. Dr. Pinto was forced to drop his research and to pick another subject.

After the Mexico City enlightenment, I returned home to Colorado with my first case of scientific frustration. My whole dental education and my first eleven years of practice were now challenged. I did know something about blood chemistry monitoring, so I began from the familiar and ventured into the unfamiliar. I ran blood tests before and after amalgam removal, and what I observed created my second case of scientific frustration. This one was far more acute than the first, for it involved patients diagnosed with incurable diseases who were improving. Hurriedly I sought to inform the leaders of dentistry that mercury was a poison. Herein I created my third case of scientific frustration, one I thought for sure was going to be terminal. And for the twenty years since then, many of my dental colleagues have been hoping it would be.

Trying to explain professional mistakes to people not familiar with the vocabulary of that profession is more than I could do alone. During the undertaking of this book, I have received aid and emotional support from three copy-editors, Marcia Kuharich, my son David, and Liza N. Burby, as well as the thousands of patients who have each contributed to my education by offering challenges. There is also my ex-wife Sharon, who now lives incognito, preferring not to be the target of those who favor the placement of amalgam. She spent many hours cogenerating parts of my original manuscript after that infamous scientific circus in Chicago in 1984—the "scientific" conference that "reaffirmed the safety of amalgam." (More about that in Chapter 4.) After seeing personal friends pretend they did not recognize us, seeing the obvious bias of the program, the broken promises, the. . . . Well, I've gotten over much of that now. That was scientific frustration number four. Thanks, Sharon, and sorry.

But what about the fellow who did the most to bring the mercury issue before the public, Tom Bearden? Bearden was with Channel 7 in Denver when he first heard about my work. He visited me in 1983 to tell me that he had heard every sham there was, and that it was useless for me to try to pull the wool over his eyes. As a result of his investigative reporting, he did two five-part series on the subject of mercury toxicity—one in 1983 and another in 1984—and won an Emmy award for his efforts. After observing my patients, he called ADA headquarters in Chicago and asked to speak with someone who was doing mercury research. He was told that so many people were doing that, it was hard to pick someone. He flew his TV crew to Chicago to observe all of this marvelous research. When he arrived, all those folks had vaporized, and he was told that the NIDR, the dental division of the National Institutes of Health (NIH) in Maryland, was doing the research. He flew on to the NIDR and asked to see all those scientists who were proving that mercury is safe in the mouth. No one there was aware of any research on mercury.

Bearden then took his findings to his television audience, and later asked the ADA if they were going to have a conference on the topic. They said yes, so he asked when. As a result of his insistence, the 1984 Chicago conference entitled the "Workshop on Biocompatibility of Dental Materials" was held. He arrived to cover the event, and was forbidden entrance. He did find one unclaimed ticket, that of Dr. Pinto, who had planned to attend. Using Dr. Pinto's ticket, he sat through the three days of presentations, and even saw the ADA's evaluation of my presentation. He bought satellite time to beam that information back to Denver. His report went something like this: "Today I read the ADA's reaction to Dr. Huggins' presentation. This is truly interesting, for his presentation is scheduled for tomorrow afternoon at two-thirty."

Bearden's reports and award-winning series were shown on many stations, and he alone informed millions of Americans that they were indeed participants in Amalgam War Three.

This book is dedicated to Tom Bearden.

Hal A. Huggins, D.D.S., M.S.
Colorado Springs, CO

*It is a well-known fact that amalgam of every known composition corrodes.*

—Schoonover and Sounder, 1941; Mateer and Reitz, 1970

*When mercury is combined with the metals used in dental amalgam, its toxic properties are made harmless.*

—American Dental Association, 1984

*The real issue is which is more important, the life of the filling or the life of the patient?*

—Hal A. Huggins, D.D.S., M.S., 1992

# Introduction

How many people are really affected by the metals in their fillings? This is the question I am asked most frequently, and it is the question I wrestled with for the first decade that I investigated the topic of toxicity. In 1984, the American Dental Association (ADA) stated in *Science Digest* that only 5 percent of the population was sensitive, and that that was too low to be significant. Someone (maybe I) pointed out that, according to statistics of epidemiology, in some cases 5 percent is considered an epidemic. If 5 percent of the population had polio or AIDS, that would be over 12 million people in the United States alone. Would that be considered insignificant by anybody other than the ADA? Strange as it seems, by the next month there were apparently many more healthy people in the United States; a new statement from the ADA showed that *only 1 percent* was sensitive. By 1989, that figure had dropped to one in 1 million; in 1991, it was back up to 3 percent. I can find no studies to support *any* of these claims, however, so I wonder how scientific they really are. My frustration involved trying to find some way to determine this other than reading hopeful opinions.

In search of the answer to this question, in 1983, I developed a patch test for mercury toxicity. A patch test involves applying a suspect substance to the skin on a small surgical pad, and observing the reaction. If the skin turns red, the patient is said to have a sensitivity to the substance. It didn't take long to find that a change in skin color was not the prime indicator that it was made out to be, however, because skin reactions are the result of allergic responses, not toxic reactions.

In working with the patch test, I found only 33 percent of the 1,000 people tested actually turned red at the site of the patch. But systemic reactions were demonstrated by *90 percent* of those tested. The term systemic refers to an internal body reaction, rather than an external reaction like a skin rash. Systemic diseases include kidney disease, lupus, multiple sclerosis (MS), diabetes, and arthritis. The systemic reactions I observed included significant changes in blood pressure, pulse, and body temperature. Since only slightly more than one-third of the reactive people actually got a red skin reaction, I concluded that the patch was not a very valid test.

The reason I stopped using the patch was that whatever people's problems were, when the patch was placed, they were apt to have a double-plus reaction in that specific area. For example, if mercury toxicity was suspected because a patient was having seizures, a patch was apt to set off seizure activity after a few hours. Migraines could be triggered, emotional upheavals generated, loss of muscle control similar to the symptoms of MS begun—enough negatives to suggest that there had to be a better way to test people, preferably something done in a test tube. I did note that my finding of 90 percent actual reactivity was far different from the ADA's 5 percent, 1 percent, 3 percent, or one in 1 million.

In 1985, at age 48, plagued by not finding answers, I went to the University of Colorado and asked Douglas Swartzendruber, Ph.D., if I could audit one of his courses in immunology. He said no, and that if I really wanted to learn something about immunology, I would have to take the prescribed courses, complete with exams. I was 52 when I obtained my Master of Science degree. My thesis, on mercury toxicity, was entitled "The Medical and Legal Implications of Components of Dental Materials." Those implications were astounding—but not as astounding as the active avoidance of confrontation of the problem by the leaders of the dental profession.

How many people are really affected by mercury toxicity? While I was at the university, I began a study that evolved into a full blown examination of immune reactivity to all of the dental components I could find. I use the term "find" advisedly, because most dental manufacturers are reluctant to let anyone know just what chemicals are in their patented materials. Many eventually became cooperative—after I signed nondisclosure agreements, and mentioned that the Occupational Safety and Health Administration (OSHA) says that we as dentists have to inform our patients of the composition of the products. In other words, if I go to jail for not informing patients, you, Mr. Manufacturer, are going to be my cellmate.

My first immune tests were a light-year ahead of the selection technique most dentists are taught in school, which is to "use whatever works best in your hands." I soon found that immunology offers many refinements if you want to look long enough and to pay enough for equipment. The most recent results of double-blind tests on over 3,500 patients shed the following light on immune reactivity of amalgam components: 95.29 percent were reactive to copper; 94.04 percent to zinc; 90.2 percent to mercury; 66.86 percent to silver; and 62.51 percent to tin.

It's interesting to note that the original patch tests showed 90 percent of the people to be reactive to mercury, and this test showed 90.2 percent. The important thing was that now there was a test that did not adversely affect patients, and that I could now test for nearly 100 dental chemicals other than mercury. This led me to find that there were many replacement dental materials that also had a negative impact on the human immune system. It is easy to jump from the frying pan into the fire, so don't just run out and replace your amalgams. I will tell you more about this in Chapter 5.

So 90.2 percent of us are reactive to mercury. So what? What is mercury toxicity anyway? What sort of reaction should we expect? Herein lies the sinister part of the problem. Not everyone reacts in the same way. If we all caught a cold when we were exposed to mercury, amalgam would have been banned decades ago. On a really basic level, the ways in which mercury attacks the body can be identified in five categories. The fifth one, miscellaneous, is actually the largest. The categories are: neurological, cardiovascular, collagen, immunological, and miscellaneous. To break these down further into the potential symptoms and the percentages of the population that experience these symptoms, following are the results of a study of 1,320 patients from whom I extracted (no pun intended) the following data.

Neurological problems encompass two divisions, motor and sensory. An example of motor problems would be tremors, while sensory might be brainfog (spaciness), short-term memory problems, or depression. The percentages of patients exhibiting these mercury-caused problems are: depression, 73.3 percent; numb fingers or toes, 67.3 percent; memory problems, 58.0 percent; frequent leg cramps, 49.1 percent; facial twitches, 52.3 percent; and jitteriness or nervousness, 38.1 percent.

As with many aspects of mercury toxicity, the term "unexplained" precedes the names of specific mercury-induced cardiovascular symptoms. Heart attacks have a specific cause. Mercury-caused problems are elusive. The percentages I have found are: unexplained chest pains, 35.6 percent, and unexplained tachycardia, 32.4 percent.

The most common problem in the collagen category is arthritis. Constant or frequent pain in the joints constitutes 35.5 percent of the symptoms in this category.

Immunological disorders are probably the most significant category, as shown by studies done in my laboratory on over 3,500 people. Over 90 percent of these people demonstrated immune reactivity. This is most often seen in what are called autoimmune diseases, or diseases in which the body's immune system attacks its own tissues. Briefly, when an atom of mercury embeds itself in a cell, the cell looks different to your immune system, and the immune cells are told to kill off that unusual-looking cell. The instances of these diseases are expanding exponentially, and, according to my observations, the combination of the new, high-copper amalgams and root canals are primary causative factors. Examples of autoimmune diseases include MS, amyotrophic lateral sclerosis (ALS or Lou Gehrig's disease), lupus erythematosus, diabetes, certain types of arthritis, and acquired immune deficiency syndrome (AIDS).

The miscellaneous category gets crowded. Some of the symptoms include: frequent urination, 64.5 percent; chronic fatigue, 63.1 percent; bloated feeling after eating, 60.6 percent; recurring constipation, 54.6 percent; ringing in the ears, 47.8 percent; metallic taste in the mouth, 38.7 percent; suicidal thoughts, 37.3 percent; and headaches after eating, 20.1

percent. The miscellaneous category also includes allergies. Many of today's food and airborne allergies seem to
show a correlation between placement of fillings and the
onset of these allergies. With allergies, just removing the
offending fillings, unfortunately, does not bring about an
alleviation of symptoms. In Chapters 7, 8, and 9, I will talk
about the steps a recovering mercury-toxic patient must
take to allay and eliminate symptoms.

How does one go about identifying mercury toxicity?
Is there a test that positively says you are mercury toxic?
Not yet, but we are on the brink of finding one. Meanwhile, there are many things we can identify that happen
to a person's blood chemistry when he or she is reacting
to mercury. Although these changes can occur in a variety
of other conditions, when they occur in conjunction with
certain symptoms, one can assemble the parts and end up
with a diagnosis.

White blood cells are quite sensitive to the presence of
components of amalgam—not just mercury, but also copper and zinc. In response to the placement of amalgam,
white cells usually go up initially. Then the differential, or
the populations of different types of white cells, moves
around in a characteristic fashion. Blood proteins, blood
sugar, cholesterol, red blood cells, oxyhemoglobin, and
liver enzymes can all do little jigs when exposed to heavy
metals. Standard tests (and many more of the sophisticated immune tests) show that all of these components
have tendencies to make unexplained moves when exposures occur to sensitized people. Heredity plays a definite
role in this, for if a person is not genetically predisposed
to develop a certain disease, all the environmental exposure in the world will not create that disease.

Obviously, it takes a lot of training and experience to
ferret out the grains of diagnosis from the chaff of interfering
chemistry. Treatment is a subject that expands every month

or two. There are so many areas affected by heavy metals that I don't know if we will ever find them all.

In the following chapters, you will learn about the history of mercury toxicity, diseases caused by mercury toxicity, testing procedures, and my treatment plan, complete with nutritional guidelines. After reading this book, you will have a good understanding of the depth of the mercury problem. May this book provide hope to those of you who have been told for so long that your problems are "all in your head."

# 1

# Amalgam
# and Its Potential
# for Destruction

In 1984, the American Dental Association (ADA), with no scientific proof, announced that 5 percent of the population (12.5 million people in the United States), was reactive to mercury and that that was insignificant. When I mentioned that 5 percent was considered epidemic by some standards, they soon changed that figure to 1 percent. I have now tested a total of over 7,000 patients, and I can show that over 90 percent of them demonstrate immune reactivity to low levels of mercury; thus the credibility battle between organizational prestige and actual tests on patients. The ADA can't lose. Neither can I. The only loser is you, the patient, who unsuspectingly allow toxic mercury materials to be placed in your mouth by dentists, who have been told by the ADA that amalgam—the generic term for silver-mercury fillings that actually contain 50 percent mercury—is safe.

## TWO AMALGAM STORIES

This is the story of my first encounter with a mercury-toxic patient:

Jan had had a thirty-minute appointment, which was not too bad since she had not had a cavity in five years. While the dentist was working on her teeth, she suddenly experienced a shooting pain in her chest and a quick short intake of breath. She wanted to hold it until the pain went away. As her eyes began to grow wider and perspiration stood out on her forehead, the dentist asked something like, "Are you all right?"

"I wasn't all right," Jan told me later, "but I didn't know what was wrong."

"Calm down," she remembered the dentist saying. "You are just uptight about being at the dentist's."

"I've never been frightened before," she complained. "It's the pain in my chest. It's awful."

She said the dentist told her she would be fine, "but the words came out of a soft cloud somewhere that surrounded me and all that was around me.

"I decided to be brave and endure—not the dentist, but the awful pain in my chest," Jan said. "I squirmed slightly in the chair and heard a whisper telling me that it couldn't possibly hurt, because he was through. I felt that I was all through, too. I wanted to close my eyes and drift off. Maybe that would stop the pain."

"I remember seeing Jan wander into the reception room where I was waiting for her," her mother said. "She had a glazed, but pained, look on her face. When I asked what was wrong, she just clutched my arm and said that she wanted to go home. The intensity of her grasp told me that I had better do just that. I sensed that a few tiny fillings could not be causing this kind of reaction, but perhaps her period was about to start and she was feeling dizzy.

"I glanced at the receptionist, but she was busy answering a telephone, and didn't seem concerned about Jan, so I brushed dentistry aside and took Jan to the car. She got into the back seat and lay down, saying something about her chest. Nothing made sense, but I took her home."

That night, Jan's mother rushed her to the emergency room of a nearby hospital. She now knew what hyperventilation was. Jan had calmed down after getting home, but then another severe pain had hit her in the chest.

"Mommy, I'm going to die," she kept reciting. Her mother had believed her, as I believed her now, while I watched this scenario that I had heard her mother tell me about over the phone. I watched as Jan quivered and cried tearless sobs, looking up from a terribly acne-pocked face. "Do something, please," Jan pleaded with me. "I'm fading."

"She never had the acne before the fillings either," her mother was saying. I wondered incredulously, She's worried about acne while her daughter is dying in front of our eyes? Obviously her mother had seen this reaction often and knew that Jan was not in fact going to die. I decided to take the cue, and to do something scientific instead of standing there paralyzed by the demonstration her mother thought I should witness. I drew Jan's blood. That was the one thing I knew something about. Perhaps the blood would tell me the secret of these recurring spells.

"What did they tell you at the hospital?" I asked.

"Which time?"

"How many times has she been to the hospital?"

"Dozens. I figured if I told you that over the phone, you wouldn't see us."

"I didn't know you were coming this time," I reminded her. I had spoken with her just once over the phone when I had told her that from the limited story she had given me, I was not the man for this job.

"You have to help Jan," her mother said. "The hospital said she was okay, the cardiologist said she was okay, the internist said she was okay, and after more than a dozen trips to the emergency room, hospitalization was recommended."

Her mother said that the final diagnosis came after X-rays, probing fingers, and an increasing feeling of fading away. What was the medical conclusion for all these problems? She had "nerves."

Her mother took her home from the hospital after that. The chest pains became more severe. Jan was sure she was going to die. There were more trips to the emergency room, more hospital tests, and more specialists. Then, when all else failed, the psychiatrist, the psychologist, the minister, and finally, the institution. Six months of pilgrimage from doctor to doctor (more than fifty in all) led to what could have been the final verdict: "Lock her up."

But you don't just lock up a winner! Her mother told me she had been voted the most popular girl in her class. She had been a cheerleader. She had been a good student. She had been a happy, charismatic kid exuding love and friendship; an outstanding child, not a person with a mental illness.

By now Jan looked as though she were physically trying to claw her heart out of her chest. I couldn't help but feel compassion for this seventeen-year-old girl who had been the rounds.

I had never seen anything like this in dental school, nor in my seventeen years of practice. I began to feel anger at the possibility that this was a variation in the vast array of problems relating to mercury toxicity. Was this a case of mercury toxicity disguised as chest pains? When the blood analysis came back, it didn't say anything to me. It would today, but in 1979 it looked "normal."

I remember that tears came to my eyes. That is not unusual. I probably went ten years without crying before I got into mercury-toxicity diagnosis. Now it was common.

At her mother's urging, I removed Jan's amalgams. She had a rough twenty-four hours. By the fourth day, she was back in school after a six-month absence. She completed two semesters of work in one and graduated with her class.

Jan was my first big exposure to the destruction of life through toxic metals, but far from my last. Today the telephone links me with that world every day. Hundreds more—in fact, 5,000 people a month—call my office for information on how to find a doctor who "believes" in toxicity. This is not easy. Today, any dentist who mentions that mercury might be a hazard is liable (under the new dentistry commandment of "ethics") to lose his license. Do you have any idea what a dentist is qualified to do to earn a living if he loses his dental license? With training, he might be able to sell used cars. Is this pressure? You bet. Fear, the best motivator, is the primary reason American dentists place nearly 1 million mercury fillings every day.

Don't ask your dentist about mercury. You might be contributing to the loss of an endangered species. Dentists have no choice but to follow the party line.

The day I met eleven-year-old Susan was December 19, 1982. She had been having seizures every fifteen minutes of her waking hours for six months. When her parents brought her to me, they said they had been told Susan had only three months to live.

I wanted her well as a Christmas present to me. I told her that. She half smiled through glazed eyes, then sank into disbelief. She had been disappointed so many times before. But I meant it. My ego was hurting. I had been telling dental groups for two years that I was going to have mercury out of dentistry by Christmas of 1982. I had failed to do this, and everyone who had heard me knew it. I had even told people to send me a Christmas card thanking me for getting rid of mercury. It was only a week until Christmas, and I estimated that nearly 1 million mercury fillings were placed on that particular December 19. There wasn't much hope of a Christmas card, but I might be able to help one young girl to have another chance. She needed that, and I needed that.

With seizures coming every fifteen minutes, we had only fourteen minutes between them to give anesthesia on both sides of her mouth, place the rubber dam, get the amalgams out, and replace them with non-mercury fillings. We did it, but then Susan had violent convulsions in the dental chair. There was no way to get her out of the chair without hurting her. One assistant put her hands on Susan's forehead and attempted to keep her head positioned in the headrest. Her father sat on her right leg and I sat on her left. Another assistant draped herself across her waist. All of us were thrown up and down like we were on a bucking bronco. We were a combined weight of over 650 pounds, and yet we were tossed into the air like rag dolls.

On December 25 she woke up. The numbness in her body was gone. Her brain was clear. She got out of bed and walked downstairs by herself! There were no more seizures. The next spring we videotaped her running the 100-yard dash in 14.8 seconds.

Later, I had a chance to hear a reaction to her improvement from the ADA. Their official comment to a Florida newspaper was, "We are not impressed." Later they were reported to say that I faked the videotape.

Where do these attitudes come from? They may be inbred. A University of Colorado School of Dentistry student called me to say he was considering dropping out of dentistry. "We were shown the video of that eleven-year-old having seizures and encouraged to jeer and laugh at it. My sister has seizures. I know those were not faked, and felt humiliated for the patient and for you. I'm not sure now that I want to be associated with such an academically dishonest profession."

A while ago, I attended a lecture at the Colorado Dental School. The guest lecturer, a specialist in dental materials, spoke of reports of teary-eyed relatives as recoveries happened. He had the whole audience of dentists (excluding an associate and myself) guffawing about such emotional involvement just because of amalgam removal.

The stories about Jan and Susan are true, but they could still be used as scripts for horror movies. I'm often asked why no one else sees these horror stories. They *are* seen by other dentists, and by other professionals as well. Clinical ecologists, who treat people who are universal reactors (allergic to everything but cotton or wood), see them all the time, but they are only just beginning to understand the implications of mercury toxicity.

These experiences, and hundreds more just like them, of lives destroyed by things beyond patient and doctor control—by things "all in your head"—are what motivated me to undertake writing this book. Reactions to mercury from "silver" fillings can occur in a documented 90.2 percent of the population. You deserve to be informed.


## WHAT IS MERCURY TOXICITY?

This question—what is mercury toxicity?—is one of the most difficult to answer, because mercury attacks the body in so many ways. Mercury kills cells by interfering with their ability to exchange oxygen, nutrients, and waste products through the cell membrane. Inside the cell, mercury destroys our genetic code, DNA, leaving us without the ability to reproduce that cell ever again. Immunologically, mercury embeds itself in a cell membrane, giving that cell the appearance of being "nonself," which is the trigger for the immune system to destroy that specific cell. With mercury in your cell membranes, the immune system will start destroying your own tissues, thus the term autoimmune disease. Examples of these are diabetes, multiple sclerosis (MS), scleroderma, and lupus.

Mercury can interfere with nerve impulse transmission, causing organs to get wrong messages. This may be related to frequent memory problems, and it can contribute to numbness and tingling of the extremities, which are notable in neurological diseases. Mercury can become attached to hormones and deactivate them, even though blood tests say that plenty of hormone is present. Many hormonal deficiencies, including thyroid, pancreas, and the sex hormones, are the result of this process.

Chronic fatigue syndrome also has a mercury component. When mercury binds to the oxygen-carrying part of hemoglobin in the blood, the hemoglobin level may look normal, but its ability to transport oxygen is hampered by mercury sitting on the transportation area. As we go through this book, you will see more detailed explanations of each of these phenomena and many more problems that fall under the heading of mercury toxicity. This is the frustrating thing about mercury toxicity: The diffuse nature of the toxin makes it very difficult to pin down.

The only scientifically recognized test that distinguishes mercury toxicity from all the other heavy metal toxicities is the urine porphyrin test. Porphyrins are the body chemicals from which hemoglobin and other energy sources are manufactured. When mercury interferes with energy production and oxygen transport, all cells in the body are affected. The porphyrins build up in the blood and excesses spill over into the urine. Certain porphyrins that appear in excess in the urine point specifically to metabolic interference by mercury. I will explain more about testing for mercury toxicity in Chapter 6.

## THE CONTROVERSY

In medicine, if a drug has one chance in 1,000 of causing an adverse reaction, the patient is informed. In dentistry, a dentist may place any number of Environmental Protection Agency (EPA)-listed toxic substances in your mouth without giving you the slightest hint of the potential side effects. Mercury, copper, nickel, beryllium, zinc, phenol, formaldehyde, diisocyanate, and acetone are just a few of the nearly 100 chemicals that are placed daily into unsuspecting patients' mouths. The ADA is fighting tooth and nail to prevent "informed consent" in dentistry. Their reasoning is that this would imply that these materials are harmful.

The automobile industry went through a similar trauma years ago when it fought against the mandatory installation of seat belts. The implication was that you could get hurt in a car. The admission of this obvious fact led to the saving of thousands of lives every year due to the presence of seat belts.

After being introduced to the problem of mercury seeping out of silver-mercury fillings by Olympio Pinto, C.D., of Rio de Janeiro in 1973, I started to observe what happened to patients' body chemistries when these mercury-laden fillings were removed. I was lecturing at the time on the subject of how to use blood chemistry to determine what nutritional intake was required to help people prevent dental decay and gum disease. As I lectured on body chemistry, I couldn't help but mention the ravages of mercury. Other dentists had begun removing amalgam from their patients and seeing the same things I was seeing. In about 10 to 15 percent of the cases, incurable conditions began to respond. (Today the figure is far higher than that, but twenty years of investigation can teach you a few things.)

At that time, I rushed to the ADA with my newfound

knowledge. The reception I received was tantamount to excommunication. I was slurred, slandered, and spit upon by people I had thought were colleagues, friends, and professional family. The scientists at the ADA, who were supposed to be doing the research we practicing dentists were paying for with our dues, were the most resistant.

Well, I was pretty naive at the time. The ADA's implication was: Just stay in the dental office, and we will handle all the politics, insurance, and research, and even tell you how to invest your money. I had bought it all. How fortunate I was to have scientists investigating all the new materials, for I certainly didn't have the time. I wouldn't know how to analyze the chemicals anyway. Since then, a former ADA employee told me what was required to obtain ADA certification of new materials. Sure, there were chemical testing requirements, but they were not as significant as a full-page ad in the *Journal of the American Dental Association* (JADA).

In 1840, dentistry fought what is now called Amalgam War One. I had just inadvertently set off Amalgam War Three, without even knowing that there had been a One and Two that had preceded me. Mercury won those wars. With the help of hundreds of dentists who are treating patients in the face of threats of license revocation, I am now making progress toward today's primary objective— generating awareness. If you knew the truth, would you choose differently? It is your body. It is your choice. Would you be among the 90.2 percent who react to mercury? How would your genetic makeup shape your reaction? Would it be significant, or pass by with only a quiver of your immune system?

In my early days of outrage, I was advised by a self-righteous professor that there was little chance of a cause-and-effect relationship between amalgam removal and disease reversal. Without proper statistical methodology, he said, there was no value to the healing I saw occurring. This was my first experience with the thought that self-serving science has failed the humanity it was designed to protect.

There seems to be a double standard here. Though I am told not to make unsubstantiated comments, it's apparently fine for the ADA to do so. The ADA has made the statement many times that there is no more of a health problem among dental personnel than there is in the general public. In an article in the June 1976 JADA, Vol. 92, the ADA quotes this portion of that statement frequently: ". . . no substantial evidence indicates that mercury intoxication is a significant problem among U.S. dental personnel." Insurance companies who have corresponded with me seem to disagree with them. And the next sentence is conspicuously missing from the ADA quotations: "However, to date, there have been no large-scale studies on which to rest such a conclusion."

I am often asked why the dental establishment does not embrace my philosophy of treatment and "approve" my work. I have tried over and over again to make excuses for my parent organization, but I am unable to do so any longer. Other concerned dentists have also appealed to the ADA, taking a conservative approach, discussing literature references, and giving good recommendations that would allow those who control the ADA to save face.

One good example of this approach was seen when the National Institute of Dental Research (NIDR)/ADA cosponsored a "Workshop on the Biocompatibility of Dental Materials" in July 1984, to which I was invited to speak. The workshop was ostensibly held for the purpose of discussing the effects of various materials used in dentistry upon the health of patients. Research was to be initiated if any of these materials (nickel, mercury, beryllium, and others) was suggested to create toxic reactions.

But the conclusions and recommendations of that workshop were written *prior* to my presentation there. Though I was told to present *only* clinical observations (not statistical or scientific documentation), I was severely criticized for failing to present documentation. It was as if the hundreds of hours spent in preparation for that presentation were wasted.

It is with anger and frustration at being unable to get the ADA even to recognize the problem that I am turning to you, the American public. I have already been criticized for this move. But I am doing it because I fear that too many of you will become ill waiting for the dental and medical establishments to do their research. Recommendations have been made by the ADA, but this means that nothing has been initiated yet. I feel it is your right to know what can happen if mercury amalgam is placed in your mouth or in the mouths of family members. In the following pages you will learn just that.

# 2
# Dynamics of
# Mercury Amalgam

*D*oes mercury pose a health problem? I can give you an unequivocal "yes" by answering these four questions:

1. Does mercury come out of fillings?

2. Does it form a toxic compound?

3. Does it form enough of this compound to produce illness?

4. Can illness be reduced or eliminated by amalgam removal?

## MERCURY *DOES* COME OUT OF FILLINGS

Amalgam is a mixture of mercury, silver, copper, tin, and zinc. Mercury comprises the largest portion (around 50 percent) and zinc the smallest (around 1 percent). Each of the close to 100 manufacturers has a slightly different formula, so the amounts of other metals vary. The copper content can vary from 3 to 30 percent, and silver from 15 to 30 percent, while tin is usually around 10 percent.

Chemical reactions normally take place between two types of chemicals. Those with positive charges react with those that have negative charges. A common example of this is when positively charged hydrogen ($H^+$) reacts with negatively charged oxygen ($O^-$) to produce $H_2O$, or water. All the components of dental amalgam are positively charged. The question is, do they actually "react" together, or do they just form a mixture that hardens?

Actually, many chemical reactions occur. More than a dozen compounds exist in amalgam. Copper joins with oxygen, mercury, chlorine, and sulfur (from foods); silver joins with tin, mercury, chlorine, copper, and combinations of all other present metals.

It is difficult to design an experiment that would produce all these potential chemical reactions in a laboratory, because the mouth contains a complex chemical environment that has yet to be duplicated in a test tube. Temperature changes; smoking cigarettes; chewing gum, ice, or tobacco; drinking hot coffee; eating salty, acidic, or bland foods; ingesting sugars; as well as having bacteria and other fillings in the mouth, all produce a constantly changing environment. Such mechanical and chemical stressors can be duplicated for no more than a few minutes at a time. But we know that there are two definite ways that mercury comes out of fillings: through electrical current and mercury vapor. A bit of history and explanation of these two mechanisms seems fitting here.

### Electrical Currents in the Mouth

Electrical current produced in the mouth is probably the single most damaging stressor, yet relatively little is known about it. Back in 1880, J.J.R. Patrick was the first to describe electrical current in the mouth. He called it oral galvanism.

In 1979, I bought an electrical current measuring device—an ammeter, similar to meters used in drugstores to check batteries—and started touching fillings. There was electrical current! Knowing very little about electrical current, and having no idea of how it would operate in the mouth, I started measuring electrical current from many different directions, hoping I would stumble onto something. It is obvious from just turning on a light switch that current flows from one place to another. Where would it flow in the mouth? Would it flow from one tooth to the one next to it, then to the one on the other side? I started recording the readings as I touched the ammeter probes to two fillings simultaneously in the same side of the mouth, then two on the left side, then cross-arch—upper right to upper left, upper right to lower left, etc. I tried every combination I could think of to see if any of them would speak to me. None of them said a thing—until I touched one probe to a filling while touching the ground probe to soft tissue, specifically the tissue under the tongue. Then I saw readings that had a mathematical relationship.

High school physics teachers like to demonstrate that if several steel ball bearings touch each other, electrical current can travel in one end and out the other end, no matter how many ball bearings there are, as long as they touch.

When a filling was touched with a meter probe, it discharged (like a flash camera), and the meter gave me a reading. If touched again a few seconds later, the filling's charge was significantly lower. Touching it a third time gave a reading that was practically unmeasurable. Given ten to twenty minutes, the charge would build up again.

Combining the discharge observations with the steel

ball bearing information, it would stand to reason that if four teeth had four fillings touching each other, a discharge of the first one would discharge all of the fillings. It sounds great; the only thing is, it didn't work that way. Each filling discharged independently. Since electrical current follows the path of least resistance, when a filling was touched, it was discharged, much as a camera flashbulb is discharged. I learned that when a filling is discharged, the current is released and runs into the body and up to the brain, which is the path with the least resistance. It doesn't discharge into the filling next to it.

Let a gold crown be placed beside an amalgam filling, though, and all kinds of electrical fury are generated. From the practical standpoint, I have seen patients who were tolerating the challenge of multiple amalgams. Then, with the addition of one gold crown, they succumbed to the autoimmune disease to which they were genetically susceptible.

Through a European research effort (G. Wranglen and J. Berendson, 1983), I learned that an electrical path exists between the filling itself and the natural fluids in the tooth under the filling. The electrical pathways that existed between the fillings and the brain, and now between the fillings and the fluids, reminded me of the famous traffic nightmare in Rome, where six streets converge into a single circular intersection with no traffic lights. Somehow the vehicles manage to enter and exit the intersection with no visible guidance. Similarly, when fillings, as electrolytes, are put into the mouth, their current must disperse. But there seemed to be no traffic light within the mouth either. The electricity dispersed with guidance no more evident than in Rome. I began to look for more details about electrical pathways generated in connection with fillings.

There are two types of electrical activity on the surface of a filling. One is like a standard battery. Two different metals in an electrolyte, a solution that can conduct electricity, will produce a current, or a flow of electrons. This is called a *bimetallic cell.* (The term "cell" refers to a minute area that produces electrical activity.)

The other type of electrical activity involves a cell that exists on a filling. It has an anything-but-obvious name: *differential aeration cell.* It sounds like something you might use in the kitchen after cutting onions, but it actually refers to electrical activity that exists between saliva in different areas that contain different amounts of oxygen. An area of saliva that is low in oxygen (closest to the filling) can react with oxygen-rich surface saliva exposed to your teeth. The resulting interreaction produces an electrical current. Either method of generating electrical current increases mercury release and subsequent exposure to the patient.

Electrical current creates two major concerns. First, it is something of an indicator of the speed of the surface chemical reactions—chemical reactions that release deadly mercury vapor. The second concern is the end result of directing electrical current into brain tissue. Might this produce pathology in the brain? Has dentistry even considered this possibility?

There is a common denominator among electrical cells. They all have both positive and negative parts. The negative part is called the *cathode.* The positive part is called the *anode, or sacrifice anode.* The term sacrifice indicates that this is the specific area from which the chemicals—in this case mercury—are being pushed out of the filling for potential absorption into the body. Now, you don't get something for nothing, so when you get electrical current, a chemical compound has to be lost; hence the term "sacrifice" anode. Something is given off there. Actually, with an amalgam, just about any of the metals can be given off. But my concern is that the largest volume of the metal sacrificed at the anode is mercury. Sacrificed so that your body can absorb it.

**Mercury Vapor**

Chemically, it looks as if mercury is able to come out of a filling. But isn't there an easy way to just measure it? Yes, it so happens that there is.

A psychologist from the University of Colorado was in my office one day, interviewing patients after their amalgams were removed. He had taken about fifty of my articles on mercury toxicity, and had put together a psychological profile of questions to determine if taking out fillings influenced a person's behavior patterns. His statement at that time was that "people process thought differently when they no longer have mercury in their mouths." At one point during the interviews he laughed, and I noticed that he had a mouth full of amalgams. I had just borrowed a Bacharach mercury detector from the Department of Public Health to test our office. Could there be enough vapor coming from all those fillings to be detected by an industrial meter? Could there be enough mercury vapor coming off to influence behavior? Probably not, I figured, but then one never knows unless he tries.

I asked the psychologist to open his mouth, placed the tube over a filling, and watched in stupefied silence as the needle went to 10, then 20, then 30, and then 50 micrograms of mercury per cubic meter of air ($mcg/m^3$). The maximum safe level of exposure for eight hours in a twenty-four-hour day, according to the Occupational Safety and Health Administration (OSHA), is 50 micrograms. At 51 mcgs, they fine the offender $10,000 and close the facility. Our professor's fillings pushed the needle up to 60, 70, and finally rested at 90 mcgs. Here was a university professor, minding his own business, yet contaminating his own body and my office with toxic mercury vapor every time he exhaled. Should OSHA fine him?

I knew that mercury came out of fillings, but I had no idea it came out *that* fast. Wilmer Eames, D.D.S., had proclaimed in JADA that amalgam emitted high vapor levels for only a few seconds. Other JADA articles had said that mercury vapor over amalgam is undetectable. How was it undetectable? By not looking!

After that my staff began to test routinely for mercury vapor above fillings and found everything from zero readings to more than double OSHA's maximum limit. One patient, after chewing gum for two minutes, exhibited a level of 300 mcg/$m^3$ over his fillings.

Other researchers since that time have reported finding high vapor levels. Independently, D.D. Gay, Ph.D. (1979), and C.W. Svare, D.D.S. (1981), registered high breath concentrations of mercury, especially after their subjects had been chewing gum.

Measuring vapor was simple enough, but what about analyzing old fillings to see whether substantial amounts of mercury are actually leaching out? Is that hard to do? Not if you have the proper equipment. Jaro Pleva, Ph.D., of Sweden (1983) analyzed a five-year-old filling and found it contained 27 percent mercury. Compare this with the average 50 percent mercury in new fillings and you can see that nearly half of the mercury had leached out in five years.

I ordered some tests from the toxicology department at Saint Francis Hospital in Colorado Springs on some amalgams of known age. They found that two fillings contained 36 percent mercury each; one was seven years old, the other, eleven. It was interesting to note that the seven-year-old amalgam had nearly double the electrical current found in the other. This suggests that mercury loss may be a function of the amount of electrical current generated by the filling.

## Copper Amalgam

As if this isn't bad enough, there is a new hazard on the

scene—high-copper amalgam. Several decades ago, copper amalgam was withdrawn from the market because of its toxicity. Its cytotoxic properties (the ability to cause death of the body's cells) are still being discussed in the *Journal of Dental Research*. In 1982, after testing several different types of amalgam, researchers found that copper amalgam yielded the most intense cytotoxicity of them all. The conclusion of the study reads this way: "Furthermore, necessity for a long-term biocompatibility test was also stressed, since the restorative materials are kept in the mouth for quite a long period once inserted."

Now copper amalgam is back. Not only is it back, but it is the fastest selling amalgam on the market today. The copper content has been changed from 20 percent (once deemed to be toxic) to 30 percent (now deemed state-of-the-art). What's bad about it as far as I am concerned is that when a patient reacts to a high-copper amalgam, his or her chances of recovery are much lower than if the amalgam of the early 1970s had been used. This is especially true in patients with neurological damage.

I had observed the difference with high-copper amalgams, but it wasn't until 1983 that I saw a hint as to why this was happening. An article that appeared in the *Scandinavian Journal of Dental Research* showed the difference between conventional amalgam and the new high-copper amalgams. The authors showed that the high-copper amalgams were so much more chemically reactive that they gave off mercury fifty times faster than conventional (3 to 6 percent copper) amalgams. Maybe that's why they are so damaging. In my opinion, high-copper amalgam certainly would have been banned immediately if our protective agencies had any concern about mercury toxicity from fillings.

You don't have to let a dentist place high-copper amalgam in your mouth. You don't have to let anyone put mercury in your molars. You particularly don't need mercury if you have any tendency toward gum disease. A Georgetown University study published in 1978 described a patient with advanced gum disease. As amalgams were removed by quadrant (one-fourth of the mouth at a time), the gum disease healed in that quadrant while continuing in quadrants where amalgam remained. After the final amalgam was removed, her whole mouth was healed of gum disease and remained healthy at the time of publication, two years after amalgam removal.

There's not much room for doubt that mercury does come out of fillings. It is easy to prove and easy to duplicate these tests.

## CORROSION *DOES* PRODUCE
## A TOXIC COMPOUND

What happens to mercury when it comes out of a filling? The next challenge concerns its toxicity. Does corrosion really *have* to produce a toxic compound to do you harm? Plain mercury, when not combined with anything, is poisonous. Isn't that bad enough? Well, it probably is, but it just so happens that mercury is highly reactive chemically. It likes to combine with biological tissue. In the mouth, mercury has the ability to combine with a carbon-hydrogen compound called a methyl group. When mercury combines with methyl groups it is called methyl mercury. Methyl mercury is 100 times more toxic than plain, elemental mercury. It is especially toxic to the brain and nerve tissue, which may explain amalgam's relationship to MS, epilepsy, and emotional disturbances.

M. Heintze, Ph.D, a researcher at the University of Lund in Sweden, showed that the process of methylation (combining a methyl group with a metal) can take place in the mouth. His 1983 publication, "Methylation of Mercury from Dental Amalgam and Mercuric Chloride by Oral Streptococci in Vitro," showed that there is a bacterium in the mouth that has a highly developed ability to methylate mercury. This bug is called *Streptococcus mutans.* According to current thought, it is the bug that is associated with dental decay. And *Strep mutans* is in everyone's mouth; you don't have to catch it.

What a situation! A bacterium that can produce deadly methyl mercury lives on the very fillings that give off mercury. Here's where the electrical discovery may play a role. We have noted that people who have more severe neurological diseases, like MS or epilepsy, or who have depression *and* suicidal thoughts, tend to have more fillings with negative electrical current. Dr. Heintze found that the conversion of mercury into super-deadly methyl mercury was enhanced by low levels of oxygen. Remember that mercury release is also increased by low oxygen levels. It makes one wonder if oral conditions might be *doubly* conducive to generating hazardous substances when amalgam is present. Another researcher, Max Osta, Ph.D., of New York University, mentioned to me that negative current provides an environment conducive to accelerated methylation.

Since the new high-copper amalgams almost always register negative charge, and *Strep mutans* is present in almost everyone's mouth, is it any wonder that a dentally restored mouth presents a real hazard to human health?

It's bad enough that methyl mercury destroys our adult tissues, but it can also cross the placental barrier and do chromosomal damage early in life. The mechanism is simple. Mercury is attracted to what are called active sites on genetic code molecules called deoxyribonucleic acid (DNA). Chemicals react with other chemicals in the body by coming together in a docking mechanism, similar to a spacecraft at a space station. When mercury is in the vicinity, it can twist a molecule a few thousandths of a degree. Now when the molecule tries to dock with another molecule, it can't, because the docking points no longer match. The body becomes like a huge hotel in which the molecule has a key that will *fit* into every door, but can't open any of them. This defect can also prevent molecular reactions from taking place. The mercury sits on a spot where other specific molecules are supposed to park. It is impossible for two things to occupy the same space at the same time, so interference in molecular reactions occurs, causing a birth defect.

Just what could be the source of this mercury? The first three months of pregnancy is the time a baby is most susceptible to mercury-produced birth defects. Mercury from the mother's fillings can cross the placental barrier and do its damage within seconds. Enough animal research has been done over the years to indicate on exactly which day of pregnancy an exposure to mercury will produce a cleft palate in test cases. Why not share this information with pregnant women? While you should check with your obstetrician before you have any dental work done, I recommend having mercury fillings removed as soon as possible.

To carry things a step further, many women have reported that amalgam removal reduced or corrected their specific amalgam-related malady. This includes the gamut of neurological, emotional, endocrine, and immune dysfunctions. Then they began to note that sexual intercourse produced the return of these same symptoms for a day or two. One woman even suggested that I test the sperm of her amalgam-laden husband for the presence of mercury. When I did, I found six micrograms of mercury per liter (mcg/l). Considering that it takes only one microgram of mercury to create disturbances, six micrograms is certainly worthy of consideration. Also, it takes but a few *atoms* of mercury to create a birth defect, and each microgram has billions of atoms. A few million molecules of mercury in one sperm could cause multiple birth defects. I have now asked many women about the problem, and the majority of those with depression and neurological problems tell me similar stories.

What about a pregnancy that occurs involving mercury from the father? How much mercury does it take for a one-celled embryo to develop a defect? One atom can create a misconnection of genes that can produce a birth defect at a specific area. Which area? There are literally millions to choose from. Some may show externally, some may not. Would an informed potential father and mother want to take this risk for their unconceived child?

Are you ready for one more step? My master's thesis is entitled, "Medical and Legal Implications of Components of Dental Materials." During my research, I had to look for other materials in amalgam that might produce birth defects and chromosomal damage. In addition to mercury, which I expected, I was surprised to find that copper, tin, and zinc could also produce birth defects.

## THERE *IS* SUFFICIENT TOXIC MATERIAL TO CAUSE DISEASE

Can enough mercury escape from amalgam to produce a toxic level? Based on an article by Thomas Eyl, M.D. (1970), blood mercury levels should not exceed 100 parts per billion (ppb). That would correspond to a daily dose not to exceed 100 micrograms of mercury. Other researchers find problems at even lower levels. R.P. Sharma and E.J. Obersteiner (1981) found that just a few micrograms severely disturb cellular function. They also found that mercury inhibits the growth of nerve fibers at much lower concentrations. "A few" sounds to me like one to ten micrograms at most. Again, this would tend to suggest that pregnant women should not have amalgam in their mouths at all—much less have a fresh batch placed.

Alfred Stock, Ph.D., of Germany (1939) and I.M. Trakhtenberg, Ph.D., of Russia (1969) identified toxicity at very low levels. Dr. Stock found problems if the air contained 2 micrograms per cubic meter (2 mcg/m$^3$) and Dr. Trakhtenberg found problems at 1 mcg/m$^3$. This is a far cry from the 100 proposed in the United States.

Whether we use 1, 2, 5, or 10 micrograms as a safe limit really doesn't matter. J. Radics, Ph.D. (1970), a European researcher, found that the average mouthful of amalgam can produce 150 micrograms of mercury in twenty-four hours. This is an average, of course, and it can be reduced by chewing ice, since cold slows the speed of chemical reactions; or increased by drinking hot coffee, since heat increases chemical reactions, or by chewing gum.

How much mercury does it take for the body to take notice? Is there enough coming out of a filling to create a problem? Come live in my Center for a few days and there will be no doubt in your mind. On a practical level, I have seen reversal of really severe disease by removal of one to three small fillings. A sixteen-year-old boy was so fatigued he could only go to school every other day. I found out that one small filling, called a pit filling, stood between him and full teenage activity. He could keep up with his peers within three weeks of the removal of the small amalgam.

As I mentioned in Chapter 1, eleven-year-old Susan was having seizures every fifteen minutes. She had only three small pit fillings. Neurologists were baffled. She had the best diagnostic workups available. But no one thought of "harmless" amalgam fillings as a potential cause. Within five days of amalgam removal, her seizures stopped, and they have not returned since.

## How Much Is too Much for a Dentist?

In the mid-1980s all dentists were sent a copy of a list of recommendations for their protection against mercury and scrap amalgam. It was published by the Council on Dental Materials and devised by the ADA. It warned of the severe hazards of the vapor coming from scrap amalgam. Scrap amalgam is the part of the filling left over when you have a filling placed. The scrap is put into a can or a box and "saved" to be returned for reclamation. The proper handling of this dangerous material that emits such harmful vapors is considered such a problem that it is recommended that dental students be taught about these hazards as well.

Here are the council's recommendations:

1. Store mercury in unbreakable, tightly sealed containers.

2. Perform all operations involving mercury over areas that have impervious and suitably lipped surfaces so as to confine and facilitate recovery of spilled mercury or amalgam.

3. Clean up any spilled mercury immediately. Droplets may be picked up with narrow tubing connected to the low-volume aspirator of the dental unit.

4. Use tightly closed capsules during amalgamation (while it is being mixed).

5. Use a *no-touch* technique for handling the amalgam.

6. Salvage all amalgam scrap and store it under water.

7. Work in well-ventilated spaces.

8. Avoid carpeting dental operatories, as decontamination is not possible.

9. Eliminate the use of mercury-containing solutions.

10. Avoid heating mercury or amalgam.

11. Use water spray and suction when grinding dental amalgam.

12. Use conventional dental amalgam compacting procedures, manual and mechanical, but do not use ultrasonic amalgam condensers.

13. Perform yearly mercury determinations on all personnel regularly employed in dental offices.

14. Have periodic mercury vapor level determinations made in operatories.

15. Alert all personnel involved in handling mercury, especially during training or indoctrination periods, of the potential hazard of mercury vapor and the necessity for observing good mercury hygiene practices.

Since scrap amalgam is the other half of the amalgam that is placed in your tooth, it seems reasonable that these recommendations should apply to you as well, if you have amalgam fillings. After all, you have the absolutely identical hazardous material in your mouth.

So let's apply these recommendations to the amalgam in your mouth:

1. Use a no-touch technique. (Keep your tongue from touching your fillings.)

2. Store in an unbreakable, tightly sealed container. (Put your head in a box.)

3. Store amalgam under water. (Keep your tongue from touching your fillings with your head in an unbreakable box submerged in water.)

4. Work in well-ventilated spaces. (Keep air circulating in your mouth while keeping your tongue from touching the amalgam with your head in an unbreakable box submerged in water.)

It makes you wonder, doesn't it? Why is the ADA highly concerned about scrap amalgam while it preaches the safety of the amalgam in your mouth? It's the same stuff.

### How Many People Are Affected?

Just how many people are affected by reactions to dental mercury? It's hard to say. Statistics are not maintained for many of these diseases, because, since they are not contagious, they do not have to be reported. Estimates are made by the relevant interest groups, but exact figures are not known.

I question the figures given for certain diseases. For example, MS is supposed to be occurring at a rate of 10,000 new cases per year. But I myself get anywhere from five to twenty calls a day from MS patients, and I'm sure that not everyone with MS knows about the Center. Also, twenty years ago if I saw an MS patient in a wheelchair, I could assume that he or she had been affected for over twenty years. Today it is common to see young women in their twenties in wheelchairs. (Occasionally I see a young male, but the vast majority of younger people with MS are female.) Some people get into wheelchairs within three years of the onset of MS. Could this be related to the new "state-of-the-art" high-copper amalgams? Is it root canals? Is it the use of antibiotics after tooth extraction? Is it all of the above?

I do know how many people are potentially affected by mercury. When I took my master's program at the University of Colorado from 1985 to 1989, I started a study of immune reactivity to dental materials. By now this has expanded to an investigation of nearly 100 chemicals, but at that time I was studying just the five toxic metals in dental amalgam, specifically mercury, copper, tin, silver, and zinc.

In a 1992 update of reactivity, I examined 3,500 patients in double-blind studies to determine what percentage of these people reacted to components of dental silver-mercury amalgam fillings. (Double-blind is a method of data gathering in which neither the subjects of the study nor the collectors of data have information as to which data go with which subject.) The results, as mentioned in the introduction, are as follows: for copper, 95.29 percent; zinc, 94.04 percent; mercury, 90.2 percent; silver, 66.86 percent; and tin, 62.51 percent. What this means is that 90.2 percent of our population has the potential to react adversely when exposed to mercury. If you have a genetic predisposition to an autoimmune disease, then your system may succumb when exposed to small amounts of mercury. If you are genetically strong, you may not get one of these diseases.

In answer to my original questions, then, it is fairly obvious that mercury *does* come out of fillings; that it *does* produce a toxic compound that is given off as the fillings corrode; and that enough of this substance *does* form to cause disease. This by itself should make us pretty sure it can cause a health problem. And when we consider the fourth element—whether illness can be alleviated by removing amalgam—there can be no doubt about mercury's deadly potential. If one of the world's most dreaded toxic compounds can be formed in the mouth and inhaled or absorbed into the body, is dentistry justified in submitting trusting patients to it on a routine basis just because it is easy to handle and it is cheap?

# 3

# Amalgam and Disease

By 1975, I had seen enough changes in what I considered medical diseases as a result of amalgam removal to believe it was time to hand over the responsibility to the medical profession and wash my hands of the issue. At that time, I told multi-board-certified medical pathologist David Bowerman, M.D., of the diseases that dental materials created. I told him I thought it was time for medicine to step in and clean up dentistry. To my amazement, he gave me a one-sentence reply: "If dentistry has created a problem, Hal, it is up to dentistry to investigate and correct the problem." Eighteen years later I am still serving that sentence.

In order to follow Dr. Bowerman's advice, I started recording changes that amalgam produced and categorizing them. I soon established five categories. They were:

1. Neurological (motor and sensory): Motor includes tremors, seizures, MS, and amyotrophic lateral sclerosis (ALS or Lou Gehrig's disease); sensory includes

Alzheimer's disease, emotional disturbances, unexplained depression, anxiety, and unprovoked suicidal thoughts.

2. Immunological: This overlaps with neurological and includes systemic lupus erythematosus, scleroderma, and rheumatoid arthritis.

3. Cardiovascular: Unexplained heart pains, high and low blood pressure, tachycardia, and irregular heartbeat are but a few in this category.

4. Collagen: This category includes osteoarthritis, but it is sometimes just referred to as collagen disease—coming unglued. (Collagen is the cementing substance between cells.)

5. Miscellaneous: This category is crowded and can include chronic fatigue, brainfog, digestive problems, and Crohn's disease.

Soon categories overlapped, new single-disease categories appeared, and I could see that the mercury multi-attack defied strict categorization. Not until the porphyrin tests concept appeared did I see the common thread. As mentioned earlier, porphyrins are body-manufactured chemicals that evolve into hemoglobin and adenosine triphosphate (ATP), the body's primary energy storage unit. *All* metabolic functions depend upon either oxygen or ATP. Mercury blocks the continuation of the reaction that turns porphyrins into hemoglobin and ATP by inhibiting the function of enzymes. In the mercury-toxic patient, therefore, *all* metabolic function is a potential target; a combination of lifestyle and genetics directs where the toxic hit will occur.

Let's take a look at the more common hits that our bodies take from mercury.

## NEUROLOGICAL DISEASES

Neurological diseases are commonly divided into two basic categories: motor and sensory. Motor problems can range in severity from occasional involuntary trembling to a completely incapacitating case of multiple sclerosis. Sensory disorders can take forms as diverse as unexplained anxiety and Alzheimer's disease. Neurological diseases are often progressive and can be disabling, which makes them frightening and traumatic for the sufferer.

Below I will describe four of these disorders that are often mercury-related.

### Multiple Sclerosis

MS is by far the biggest portion of my practice. Is it a dental disease? It certainly appears to be. Most physicians scoff at the idea that there is mercury in dental fillings, saying, "Maybe they used it 100 years ago, but I don't believe that dentistry would be foolish enough to place mercury in people's mouths today." I appreciate their exalted opinion of dentists, but if 100,000 of the 140,000 dentists in the United States place nine fillings per day each—about three hours' worth of work—that is 900,000 mercury fillings per day, which is probably a pretty conservative estimate.

Douglas Swartzendruber, Ph.D., an experimental pathologist at the University of Colorado, recently compiled articles from the scientific literature relating MS not only to mercury in general, but specifically to mercury from dental fillings. According to Dr. Swartzendruber's assessment of these articles:

As early as 1966 Dr. E. Baasch published in the *Archives of Neurology and Psychiatry* that epidemiologic evidence supported an environmental agent rather than an infectious agent as being the cause of MS. He proposed that mercury, the predominant exposure being from amalgam fillings, was the primary etiologic agent for MS, the pathophysiology being a neurologic response. In great detail he demonstrated that facts concerning the geographical and age distribution, pathological development and symptomatology of MS are consistent with amalgams as the primary cause of the disease.

Further, Dr. Swartzendruber found that a hypothesis presented in 1983 by Theodore Ingalls, M.D., in the *American Journal of Forensic Medicine and Pathology* proposed that the seepage of mercury from root canals or amalgam fillings might lead to MS in middle age. Based on his own personal experience, he proposed a correlation between unilateral MS symptomatology (symptoms affecting one side of the body) and amalgam-filled teeth on that side of the mouth. He also reexamined the extensive epidemiological data that showed a direct, linear correlation between death rates from MS and numbers of decayed, missing, and filled teeth in the United States and other countries. Dr. Ingalls suggested that investigators studying the causes of MS should carefully examine a patient's dental history. Later, in 1986, Dr. Ingalls published data (in the same journal) supporting his hypothesis and clearly demonstrating endemic clustering of MS in time and space, over a fifty-year time span, that could be directly correlated to exposure to mercury.

I was fortunate enough to meet Dr. Ingalls before his death from MS. He showed the pictures of his root-canaled tooth, which was filled with a mercury filling at the root tip. This amalgam was placed just prior to the onset of his MS. He showed me photographic evidence of the amalgam tattoo, or embedded amalgam, that had appeared on his gums where the mercury implant surgery had been performed. He was one of the kindest, most compassionate men I have ever met, and his primary desire was to stop the placement of mercury fillings.

Actually, Dr. Ingalls had had a twofold opportunity to contract MS. Not only did he have immunoreactive mercury in his mouth, but as I mentioned, he had had a root canal. Root canals are also immunoreactive, and in many cases more vicious than mercury.

The Multiple Sclerosis Society has been averse to looking into this situation. It is almost as if the organization wants to be *looking* for a cause and cure for this disease, but not to *find* one. They have actively campaigned against looking into the mercury issue. They have sent out letters stating that they have thoroughly checked the literature and have found no correlation between amalgam and MS. Yet Dr. Swartzendruber has written about twenty reference articles, in addition to the one I quoted, that show this relationship to be valid.

On a personal basis, the first patient to be treated in the Huggins Diagnostic Center in 1991 was Chuck Rekoske, former chairman of the Kansas MS Society. He had MS, and he did very well following treatment and amalgam removal. He got to the point where he could play three sets of tennis each day with his teenage son—and beat him. Unfortunately, he overdid it and crashed. He is now trying to pick up the pieces again, but there is another point to the story. After his improvement, he was asked by the national society to resign his post for reasons of "conflict of interest." He was recommending amalgam removal. Chuck is an interesting fellow. He declined to resign.

## Amyotrophic Lateral Sclerosis

A comparatively new disease, amyotrophic lateral sclerosis, or ALS, has come on the scene in vast numbers. It is also known as Lou Gehrig's disease. This is the most vicious disease I have confronted. It is similar to MS in that it attacks the nervous system, but it does so with the vengeance of a feeding shark. Many times it attacks the voice before the motor functions of moving hands, legs, and feet that most of us take for granted. Its duration from start to finish (death) is around three years.

There are a lot of diseases that destroy a person bit by bit, but for some reason, this one really gets to me. From 1973 until 1990, my treatment achieved no response in ALS patients, yet I could see all the chemical earmarks that suggested it was an autoimmune disease of dental origin. Finally, in early 1991, I hit upon a new button that could give a wake-up call for nerves and muscles in the ALS patient—cavitations. This is my term for a literal "hole in your head."

When teeth are removed, the periodontal ligament (a membrane that attaches the tooth to the bone) is usually left in the socket. I now compare this membrane to the afterbirth that is delivered after a baby is born. If the afterbirth is left in, the mother will probably die. When the periodontal ligament is left in, the patient does not die, but neither does the socket area completely heal. Bone cells will naturally grow to connect with other bone cells after tooth removal—providing they can communicate with each other. If the periodontal ligament is left in the socket, however, bone cells look out and see the ligament, so they do not attempt to "heal" by growing to find other bone cells.

In these cases, I have found that the top of the socket seals over with two or three millimeters (mm) of bone; under that, a hole remains. This bony hole is usually lined with chronic inflammatory lymphocytes, which are the cells of autoimmune disease, and some strange cells that took a while to identify. They turned out to be monocytes (large white blood cells with a single nucleus) that had somehow evolved three more nuclei, so that they now had a total of four nuclei. This type of cellular change can occur in an extremely toxic environment.

The significant discovery I made is that if these cavitations are opened and the periodontal ligament is removed (a five-minute procedure), ALS patients respond. Now, these people did not hop out of their wheelchairs and run the 100-yard dash, but their mobility improved, their voices improved, and their attitudes improved. These changes indicated that healing could take place, and that ALS is not an entirely nonresponsive disease. Some patients who received very early treatment have returned to near normal—I say near because these people will never be able to play three sets of tennis a day or overtax their damaged immune systems. But their life expectancy is increased by eighteen months to three years.

According to Dr. Swartzendruber's literature findings:

> The accumulation of mercury from amalgam in the CNS [central nervous system] is an important connection to the etiology of neurologic disorders such as multiple sclerosis and amyotrophic lateral sclerosis. The neurotoxicity of mercury has been long known, mercury induced neuropathology well-described, and the mechanisms of toxicity have been studied in great detail. It has also been documented by at least five independent studies that chronic exposure to mercury is an etiologic agent in the ALS syndrome. It has been clearly demonstrated that mercury from amalgam accumulates in the brain and CNS and autopsy studies show that the level of mercury in the brain linearly correlated

with the number of amalgam surfaces on fillings. Concentrations in the tissues reached as high as 120 nanograms per gram of tissue.

Based on Dr. Swartzendruber's findings, I would say that mercury toxicity is definitely related to ALS.

## Parkinson's Disease

Parkinson's disease, another neurological manifestation of heavy metal toxicity, now also responds to treatment. Prior to 1990, I felt that I could recognize all the imbalances involved, and that I knew how to correct each one of them. There was only one problem—the treatment didn't work. After finding the cavitation connection, Parkinson's began to respond beautifully. I found this especially rewarding, for Parkinson's is what claimed my mother, and I have always had a personal vendetta against the disease.

## Alzheimer's Disease

Alzheimer's disease really deserves the dual masks of theater award. Many of my experiences with these patients have been strangely humorous, while others have been truly tragic. Despite the theatrics, it is another one of those diseases that appears to be in the "it didn't have to happen" category. Clearly mercury removal affects these people, although not always within a few days. It can take weeks or months, although occasionally I see significant changes within the two-week stay that they have with me.

One minister's wife had not spoken a word for fourteen years. Ten days after amalgam removal she mumbled something. Shocked, the minister said, "What did you say?"

"Nothing," she shouted at him.

The minister called a couple of months ago and said, "Can you put maybe just one or two amalgams back in her? She hasn't stopped talking for three months. I can't get a word in edgewise."

Not all cases turn out that well, but ask Tom Warren about it. He is the author of *Beating Alzheimer's*. His CAT scan says that the lesions on his brain are gone. It took a few years, but he is very active in trying to rid the world of mercury because of what it did to him and fellow Alzheimer's patients.

Strangely, it was Alzheimer's that taught me about coloring agents in dentures. Several patients in a row had had dentures, and I decided to investigate the coloring agents in denture acrylic. It turns out that the pink coloring agents are cadmium sulfate and *mercury sulfate*. Today I make all plastic appliances, including dentures, out of clear acrylic. Sometimes I tint the first three millimeters of gum tissue over the upper front teeth with pink, because they certainly do look better. I figure that is one one-thousandth of the acrylic in a denture, and I have been getting away with it.

Not all Alzheimer's patients respond, and they certainly don't recover overnight, though of course that is what families would like to see. The family is frequently the most difficult part of the disease to treat. The patient just kind of wanders around in and out of other people's lives. Patients really require around-the-clock "baby-sitting" that the family must provide.

Three months after treatment, it usually becomes obvious if an improvement is going to occur. Six months is better than three, and nine months is better than six. So it continues for years. It is not always dramatic, but it can be satisfying to a not-overly-demanding family. After two years, one woman got a driver's license. She used to get lost in the kitchen in her own home. One dentist couldn't find the office he had practiced in for forty years. He is now back at work. And he doesn't place amalgams anymore.

Alzheimer's is really tough to treat because each step is so critical and the wandering mind of the patient is not 100-percent cooperative. A whole center devoted to the treatment could be highly successful if staffed by lots of caring, slow-moving, patient, well-trained, psychologically oriented personnel. I have seen successes, but it takes a lot of time and underwriting by my office. I have also heard of people rushing the Alzheimer's patient to a dentist and having all fillings removed at once with no precautions. Results have been less than desirable without safeguards such as blood tests, nutrition and supplementation, intravenous support, use of the rubber dam, electrical sequential removal, use of compatible dental materials, and avoidance of the seven–fourteen–twenty-one–day immune cycle.

## IMMUNOLOGICAL DISEASES

Autoimmune disease, in its simplest form, means self-destruction by the immune system. White blood cells (your immune system) are programmed to keep up minute-by-minute surveillance of every cell in your body. The system recognizes only two things: self, which is you, and nonself, which is anything else. It determines this by looking for a five-protein code on the surface of each cell. If the code is there, it moves on. If the code has been altered in any way (such as by the addition of an atom of mercury), then the surveillance system identifies the cell as nonself and goes into its normal routine to destroy the invader. Looking at the situation from this standpoint, the immune system is not the bad guy that it is sometimes made out to be in these diseases, but it is performing its role of eliminating all that is not self. Sure, they are self cells as far as you are concerned, for they may be in your kidney (as in lupus), or joints (as in arthritis), or nervous system (as in MS), but as far as the immune system is concerned, it is abnormal tissue. Your code plus an atom of mercury signifies nonself by definition.

The usual medical solution in autoimmune diseases is to stop the immune system. Another viable approach might be to stop the invasion of mercury that is causing the immune system to destroy the body's own tissues.

This category also includes airborne and food allergies. The reason for this is that heavy metals frequently disturb cell membranes in such a manner that the exchange of oxygen, nutrients, manufactured proteins, and the elimination of waste products become jumbled. Just removing the offending metals will rarely correct the damage in these people. Here is where I found the value of taking a multidisciplinary approach to patient care. This applies to MS as well.

### Arthritis

Rheumatoid arthritis is an autoimmune disease that doesn't necessarily shorten life, but the affected often wish it would. I frequently chide the arthritic that if the disease killed you in a couple of years, you could put up with it. But hurting a little bit more each day for thirty years is harder to take. Only the arthritic laughs, for only he really knows what it is like to live with pain associated with each motion twenty-four hours a day.

Mercury's role here is similar to its role in all other autoimmune diseases. With the addition of an atom of mercury to a molecule of joint tissue, the immune system identifies the tissue as nonself, or foreign, and proceeds to destroy it.

When amalgams are removed, the pain of arthritis can be drastically reduced within a few days, but it can come back if you are not disciplined in following the proper lifestyle. Removal of amalgam can give the immune system a glorious stimulation for a few days, but it settles down and then a patient's lifestyle can upset it easily. Everyday creature comforts—a cup of coffee, a bite of fish, or an orange—are sometimes the worst reactivators of arthritis. Nutrition is extremely important to the maintenance of a recovering immune system. Violation of the prescribed diet is the single most obvious factor in the return of autoimmune disease. I will explain this further in Chapter 7.

## Lupus

Systemic lupus erythematosus is a disease you can measure. There is an antibody present in the blood called the antinuclear antibody (ANA). Measurement of this antibody in the blood is generally used as an indicator of the severity of lupus.

Many autoimmune diseases don't have a yardstick, but lupus is measured by the *antibody titer*. Titration is a method of diluting a test sample to see how many dilutions are required before no more reactions occur. It would be like taking a sample of milk and diluting it with an equal amount of water and looking to see if the white cloudiness of milk is still there. This would be a 1 to 1, or 1:1, dilution, and if you could still see the cloudiness of the milk, the reaction would be called positive at a 1:1 titer.

Generally, the higher the titer, the worse the condition. In lupus, from what my patients tell me, a titer of 1:160 is considered a pretty terminal sentence. One of my patients was told that nothing could be done for her when she was diagnosed as having lupus. She went home from the doctor's office, pulled the covers over her head, and cried for two days, thinking she would die at any moment. Her titer was 1:160. After two months of nagging by her daughter, she went through my program. That was last year. Today she has a 0 titer, but still remembers the nightmares of those two months.

Rhonda Myers just had an eight-pound baby boy. About three years ago, she had a titer of 1:6400. Her titer came down to 0 in six weeks. I have not seen that happen so swiftly since then, but it suggests that there are buttons out there that do make a difference when you can find and push them. Two years later, Rhonda wanted to get pregnant. Pregnancy is tough on the immune system after you have had an autoimmune disease, and I advised against this one. She and her husband wanted to try anyway. They promised to watch her diet with extreme diligence—which they did—and she delivered a healthy son, without complications to herself or the child.

## SYMPTOMS

Diseases are one thing, symptoms are another. Symptoms are annoying disorders that may be signs of, or may lead to, a disease. For instance, a runny nose and a cough are symptoms; bronchitis and pneumonia are diseases. A problem like chronic fatigue syndrome is more of a bundle of symptoms than a disease, but it is very irritating if you have a job to perform or a family to raise. Table 3.1 lists some of the more common symptoms experienced by 1,320 patients who were studied for frequency of symptoms suspected to be of dental origin.

**Table 3.1** Percentage of 1,320 Patients Who Experienced
Symptoms of Suspected Reactions to Dental Materials

| Symptom | Percentage |
| --- | --- |
| Unexplained irritability | 73.3 |
| Constant or very frequent periods of depression | 72.0 |
| Numbness and tingling in extremities | 67.3 |
| Frequent urination during the night | 64.5 |
| Unexplained chronic fatigue | 63.1 |
| Cold hands and feet, even in moderate or warm weather | 62.6 |
| Bloated feeling most of the time | 60.6 |
| Difficulty with short-term memory | 58.0 |
| Sudden, unexplained, or unprovoked anger | 55.5 |
| Constipation on a regular basis | 54.6 |
| Difficulty in making even simple decisions | 54.2 |
| Tremors or shakes of hands, feet, head, etc. | 52.3 |
| Twitching of face and other muscles | 52.3 |
| Frequent leg cramps | 49.1 |
| Constant or frequent ringing or noise in ears | 47.8 |
| Shortness of breath | 43.1 |
| Frequent or recurring heartburn | 42.5 |
| Excessive itching | 40.8 |
| Unexplained rashes, skin irritation | 40.4 |
| Constant or frequent metallic taste in mouth | 38.7 |
| Jumpiness, jitteriness, and nervousness | 38.1 |
| Constant death wish or suicidal intent | 37.3 |
| Frequent insomnia | 36.4 |
| Unexplained chest pains | 35.6 |
| Constant or frequent pain in joints | 35.5 |
| Tachycardia | 32.4 |
| Unexplained fluid retention | 28.2 |
| Burning sensation on the tongue | 20.8 |
| Headaches just after eating | 20.1 |
| Frequent diarrhea | 14.9 |

In addition, there may be a link between mercury in the body and the successful treatment of bacterial infection. According to a publication by Dr. Anne Summers of the University of Georgia, mercury from amalgam fillings may be a significant factor in explaining why many people are becoming antibiotic resistant. In a study on monkeys, Dr. Summers found what has been known for years: Mercury alters the effectiveness of antibiotics.

Five weeks after silver-mercury amalgams were placed in monkeys, the bacteria in their intestines became resistant to mercury. Simultaneously, they became resistant to some of the most commonly used antibiotics, including penicillin, streptomycin, kanamycin, and tetracycline.

The resistance action here involves the action of bacteria when exposed to mercury. Most cells would die upon this exposure, but certain bacteria are able to defend themselves by picking up an extra piece of DNA from surrounding tissues and attaching it to their own DNA. Such an addition is called a *plasmid*. With the addition of the plasmid, the bacteria become resistant to mercury, and no longer take the invading inorganic form of mercury and convert it to an organic, excretable form. This gives the bacteria's host an additional dose of methyl mercury, which is highly toxic to many systems in the body. The nervous and reproductive systems are particularly sensitive to this process.

The new bacteria form (the original one plus the plasmid) has other changed metabolic characteristics, too. It is now resistant to antibiotics that would normally kill it. And the new bacterial form is able to reproduce the plasmid along with its own DNA, so it will always retain its resistance to certain antibiotics. This is one of the factors that has led to the development of the "antibiotic-of-the-month club" we have seen in the past several decades. As you can see, the ways in which mercury can affect our bodies are practically unlimited.

It is easy to understand the confusion about whether or not to use mercury in the mid- to late-1800s, when chemical testing and patient tracking were minimally available. With today's technology, the existence of well-financed foundations, and a plethora of research scientists studying multiple ramifications of disease, it is difficult to understand how so much that is obvious is missed. Is science so narrowly focused that it cannot see? Has science failed us? And what about the fact that many conditions are obviously improved by amalgam removal? Why do dental "leaders" continue to actively campaign against removing toxic substances even though we know this can relieve human suffering? Why do they continue to cry, "Science doesn't prove!" instead of exercising a little compassion for their fellow humans? I don't know. My only answer is to continue to generate awareness.

# 4

# The Amalgam Wars

*T*eeth have been filled with metals for centuries. We have evidence of gold bands being used to hold in an extracted tooth (similar to today's bridgework) dating back to Phoenician times. In the early 1800s, a mixture of powdered silver and mercury was used to fill teeth. It was cheaper than gold and easier to place. (The ADA uses the same reasoning to excuse today's usage.) The mixture used in the 1800s expanded upon setting, and very painfully split some teeth in two. Because of this, and because of the poisonous aspect, some dentists objected to its use, while others praised it due to its cheapness. Thus began the most significant dentistry war ever started—the war about the use of amalgam.

Mercury is poisonous. Any high school kid knows that. So how is it that our nation's dentists (educated for eight rigorous years beyond high school) can daily, in good conscience, fill their patients' teeth with an amalgam consisting of approximately 50 percent mercury? It is a result of ceaseless misinformation combined with misplaced trust.

Dentists have been taught that mercury stays within a filling and does not come out. When a dentist looks to the professional literature for information about mercury, he is apt to find statements like this one from an editorial in the *Journal of the American Dental Association* (JADA, Vol. 82, March 1971), in answer to the question, Are amalgam fillings hazardous to the patient?: "The answer is an unqualified no. Study after study shows the patient undergoes no risk . . . the dentist, yes, but the hazard can be reduced to practically zero." No one is likely to challenge a statement based on "study after study."

Dental journals condense many months of research into a few pages. The dentist can thus gain years of experience from technical trade journals. These are called refereed journals. This term means that experts in specific subspecialty fields have reviewed and scrutinized the articles for truth and honesty. Dentists rely on this implied integrity, and they tend to believe what they read in these publications without challenge, because dentistry is thought to be a highly ethical profession.

Yet looking back at that JADA quotation now, after twenty years of investigation into mercury toxicity, I note that these "studies" were not referenced. In the thousands of articles I have collected on mercury in the body, I have not been able to find even one that would support the claim that mercury is harmless to the patient. Nonetheless, this statement stands unchallenged by dentistry in general.

The same issue of JADA contained an article that made a similar claim: "The amount of mercury vapor emitted from an amalgam is undetectable." Again, there was no substantiation, just a statement. Information like this tends to lull dentists into thinking that they are working with a material that is unquestionably safe for their patients. It may be dangerous in all other areas, but it is completely safe in the mouth.

Yet in contrast to this, dentists are required to read

articles that suggest minimizing their own risk and the danger to their personnel by using the no-touch technique described in Chapter 2. They are cautioned to avoid touching amalgam with their fingers, and to get rid of scrap amalgam because it is *dangerous* to the dentist.

If mercury is so safe in your mouth and so dangerous in your office, then Jerry Timm, D.D.S., was right when he said, in a letter to the editor that appeared in the April 26, 1982 issue of the ADA newsletter, that the dental association is telling us that "the only safe place to store amalgam is in the mouth."

In Chapter 2, I discussed the composition of amalgam. If the 50 percent that is mercury stayed tightly bound in the amalgam filling, as dentists are taught, then five- or ten-year-old fillings would still contain that 50 percent mercury. They don't. Actual tests have shown that they contain 25 to 35 percent mercury by that time. And as I mentioned earlier, some twenty-year-old fillings have been shown by Dr. Pleva to contain less than 5 percent mercury.

Some people suggest that fillings should therefore become less of a problem the older they get. "No," say the allergy doctors. "The more often you are exposed to a substance, the more apt you are to become allergic to it." In addition to this factor, mercury is a cumulative poison.

## AMALGAM WAR ONE

Is mercury toxicity a new topic? Hardly. It has been debated in dental circles since the 1830s. According to W.H.C. McGehee, amalgam was first introduced in England in 1819 by a man named Bell and later used by a dentist named Traveau, who placed it commercially in Paris in 1826.

In the late 1820s, amalgam was introduced to America as a cheaper substitute for the only filling material used at that time, gold. Dentists began to quarrel about its use right away. Mechanically, the first amalgams were inferior to today's, and tended to expand as they reacted with saliva. As I mentioned, some teeth actually split as the amalgam expanded. You can imagine the pain people experienced as their fillings slowly split their teeth apart. Dentists who placed gold immediately censured their colleagues for such practices. They also pointed out the poisonous aspects of mercury.

Amalgam placers said that the gold placers were only interested in money, and were in essence denying services to lower income patients. On the battle raged, until it became the Amalgam War. Articles began to appear in the dental literature. The Amalgam War became an academic conflict. The emotional pitch of the nineteenth-century conflict is evident in some of the titles of the academic onslaughts:

- "Death Caused by Swallowing Large Amalgam Filling" (*Advertiser*, Dental, 1881,13).

- "Diseased Eyes and Amalgam Fillings" (S. Clerotica, *American Dental Review*, I, 1858, 68–69).

- "Mercurial Necrosis Resulting from Amalgam Fillings" (J.Y. Tuthill, *American Journal of Dental Science*, XXXIII, 3rd Series, 1899-1900, 97–108).

- "A Shameful Case of Malpractice (Amalgam Filling)" (George H. Weagant, *Dental Items of Interest*, VIII, 1886, 73–74).

- "Irritation of the Larynx Caused by an Amalgam Filling" (Otto E. Inglis, *Stomatologist*, IV, 1900, 155).

The dental community became polarized into two camps: those who abhorred amalgam, and those who advertised it heavily. Irreconcilable differences between the two camps undermined the foundation of the National Association of Dental Surgeons, and soon dentistry was without a professional organization.

In 1899, a new organization came into existence—the American Dental Association. It endorsed amalgam and grew to become the ADA of today. It still endorses amalgam, but the old Amalgam War veterans continue to whisper to today's consciousness.

## AMALGAM WAR TWO

The Amalgam War was reasonably quiet as a new generation of dentists came into practice believing that amalgam was the material of choice for the majority of fillings. Then, in the 1920s, an intermediate skirmish began in Europe. This was later dubbed Amalgam War Two. Dr. Alfred Stock, a prominent German chemist, led the fight, but he didn't consider it a war. He was just reporting what he thought was valuable scientific evidence that mercury was poisonous and that it leached out of fillings, producing diseases in many folks. He published over thirty articles condemning the use of amalgam. His research methods were surprisingly accurate; they rival the most sophisticated techniques of the 1990s. He gained headway in drawing attention to diseases that were stimulated by mercury leaching out of fillings. He had become suspicious that mercury was the source of his own myriad of medical problems and had his amalgams removed. When his medical problems improved as a result of amalgam removal, he then diagnosed many friends' problems and encouraged them to have their amalgams removed. Finally, the European medical community gave credence to his findings and he gained academic, as well as public, support. Then the dental community started a program to discredit him and gave him an enormous amount of grief.

Dr. Stock became discouraged and lost his drive in his research when his laboratory and most of his records were destroyed by a bombing raid in World War II. World War II ended Amalgam War Two, and Dr. Stock died in near obscurity.

After that, very little was heard about amalgam for three decades. I was certainly unaware of mercury hazards during my dental training in the late 1950s and early 1960s. As students, we mixed eight parts of mercury with five parts of powdered metal, placed the soupy mixture in a squeeze cloth, and twisted the cloth to "express" out the excess mercury. The excess mercury would fall onto a metal tray and roll into a reservoir of mercury. Some of the liquid mercury would hit the metal tray and splash onto the floor. Thousands of tiny droplets would scatter across the clinic floor to find new homes in cracks, equipment, and shoes. According to figures published years later, only 20 percent of the mercury dispensed left the clinic in patients' mouths.

## AMALGAM WAR THREE

I suppose we could say that Amalgam War Three started in Mexico City in 1973. At least the soldiers were introduced to each other at that time. I had spoken before the International Academy of Gnathology on how balancing body chemistry (my primary subject of interest at that time) could increase bone density and reduce gum disease. Healthy bones and gums can greatly aid the efforts of gnathology, the science of reconstructing tooth surfaces (usually with gold or porcelain crowns) according to the dictates of a complex instrument that records the forward, backward, and side-to-side movements of the jaw. I pointed out several blood chemistry abnormalities that would not respond to treatment, and casually mentioned that I did not know why.

That gap in my knowledge was soon filled, as Dr. Olympio Pinto came up to me after my presentation. "Those nonresponsive areas are easy to explain," he began. "They are due to sulfhydryl blockage by mercury leaching out of amalgam fillings." I wasn't too sure what sulfhydryl blockage was, but at the time I was still secure in my belief that amalgam was a stable compound.

"Why? Mercury doesn't come out of amalgam," I began, and then muttered something about alpha phase, gamma phase, and other terms I mimicked from my dental school professors. I could see that I wasn't having much impact on this man from Brazil. How was I to know that I was talking to one of the world's authorities on mercury toxicity?

Dr. Pinto explained that his parents had both been dentists. His father had attended a conference in the 1920s at which a speaker had condemned mercury. The elder Pinto remembered this a while later when he was asked to treat a child dying of leukemia. Her biggest complaint was that her gums hurt. He removed her amalgams quietly, and the terminally ill child responded within a few days. "Spontaneous remission!" announced the medical profession. Pinto responded by telling the physician he had removed the amalgams. There was a pecking order at that time, just as there is today, in the health professions. He was academically whiplashed and made to feel inferior and foolish. This was standard procedure. So Pinto quietly replaced an amalgam in the little girl, then told the doctor to watch for a recurrence of the leukemia the next day. There was a recurrence. He removed it, of course, and the child recovered again.

"Then there was the case of Hodgkin's disease," Dr. Pinto continued.

"Hodgkin's?" I retorted. "Wait a minute. You're talking about heavies. Medical diseases! Real diseases! Not allergic reactions."

Dr. Pinto quietly proceeded with diseases and dates. "This type of lymphoma was not noted until 1832, a short time after amalgam was introduced in the area where the disease was discovered. The first amalgam to be placed in an African-American was in 1904. Sickle-cell anemia was noted to move out of the rare in 1906."

"But pathologists weren't very smart then," I challenged. Later I found that some of the most brilliant pathologists the world has ever known were alive then. I also learned that sickle cells are not difficult to identify.

I argued that these could be spontaneous coincidences, that there were no double-blind studies, that. . . . I sputtered while he continued to deluge me with anecdotes. Then he began quoting scientific literature.

"Where did you come up with that information?" I finally asked.

"I was taking a master's degree at Georgetown University. Mercury toxicity was my topic. I compiled the largest bibliography on mercury toxicity that probably existed on the planet at that time," he answered.

"When was your thesis published?" I asked.

"It never was. The National Institute of Dental Research—part of the National Institutes of Health—found out about my project and forced the university to have me stopped. I had a choice of returning to Brazil or changing my topic. I had no choice, but I still have the materials."

Dr. Pinto sent me his material. I was captivated by it and suggested that it be published. He was still discouraged by his treatment by Americans and declined to put any more time into the subject, but encouraged me to assemble it if I wanted to. The result of many intercontinental conversations was published in 1976, under the title "Mercury Poisoning in America."

By the end of my first two hours with Dr. Pinto, I had made a solemn personal vow. I would never mention these findings to a dental group. I kept that vow with an agonized, haunting feeling that someday the secret would slip out. And it did, just three weeks later, while I was lecturing to an especially cordial group in the South.

"Would you fellows like to hear something really way out?" I heard myself say. As I told the mercury story, one member of the audience paled. He had had Hodgkin's and had been told his case was terminal. His amalgams were removed during a dental study club educational project and his diagnosed Hodgkin's had gone into *spontaneous* remission. That was about twelve years prior to my presentation. I felt a cold chill spread from my neck outward to my arms, legs, feet, and hands. My eyes became cloudy. It was then that I truly experienced the start of Amalgam War Three.

The years from 1973 through 1979 were frustrating ones. Success would peek through the muddled chemistries about once every three to six months. Then it would disappear, leaving no hope that it would ever reappear. I met with many more failures than successes in my attempts to be another Dr. Pinto. I continued to mention the problem as I lectured on body chemistry. Everyone thought it was interesting, but in private would let me in on certain "secrets." These confidential comments went like this: "If mercury were really a problem, the ADA would have found it out 100 years ago and eliminated it." "The Food and Drug Administration (FDA) would certainly not allow such a substance to be used. They are here to protect the health of the public." "Congress would certainly legislate sanctions against mercury if it were a problem." "The American Medical Association (AMA) monitors everything related to health. They would surely spot any problems that might have arisen."

I would ask them, "If we are protected, how do you explain the one case in ten or fifteen of mine that *has* responded?" Their answer was simple—spontaneous remission!

I wanted to quit. I prefer success to failure, and certainly the scales were tilted. I lost more than I won. My colleagues were interested, but not supportive. The successes—like the cessation of chronic headaches, the lifting of brainfog, and feelings returning to the fingers of MS patients—were uplifting, but the times when nothing happened made me feel I might be wrong. The time spent, the financial drain, the emotional drain, and the friendships that dissolved were easy to put on the scales. I was teaching how to balance chemistry, while I was personally living a totally unbalanced life. I've been asked many times, "Why did you continue?" I have an honest answer: I don't know.

Then came 1979. That was the year when pieces of the puzzle began to come together and actually fit. What a delightful year that was. There were more cases to attempt, and a higher percentage of successes. Electrical current became the biggest breakthrough. I found that if I removed negative current fillings first, the changes in white blood cells were more beneficial, and symptoms began to respond more often. The mercury vapor meter appeared, and it took only two minutes to find that there was adequate vapor coming off of fillings to be measured with an industrial meter. This was proof. The ADA was not impressed. But the meter still showed that vapor was coming off much faster than I had imagined possible. Al Belian, D.D.S., told me about iron binding sites. These hold life-sustaining oxygen on the hemoglobin. Eventually this explained part of chronic fatigue syndrome. Dr. Pinto sent me a videotape of what happens to red and white blood cells when you eat foods that you should not. It was amazing to watch cells change from one form to another (a process known as pleomorphic changes). This is rather like a worm crawling into one end of a cocoon, and crawling out the other end as a butterfly. Foods are important in the healing process. This video showed why. This also led to the development of the Lazerview microscope some fourteen years later, which is a microscope that can see abnormal living cells and work with computer technology to identify them. The electron microscope is more powerful, but can be used to examine only dead tissue. I wondered what the Lazerview would bring.

These were exciting years. I was lecturing more and describing what I was seeing to more doctors who were getting interested in trying this for themselves. New disorders were responding, like unexplained fatigue, unexplained depression, unexplained chest pains (the key word in mercury toxicity seems to be "unexplained"). Digestive problems due to alteration of "gut bugs"—the friendly bacteria in the digestive tract that aid in the digestion of carbohydrates, protein, and fat—became evident.

My success rate went up to 50, 60, and 70 percent. Elation over patient improvements was evident in my whole staff. Phone calls were approaching twenty to thirty a day. The mail was heavier, interest was expanding, workdays were becoming longer, financial productivity was dropping as I tried to satisfy unrealistic requests from the public and professionals, and accounting figures began to show red ink. Due to lecture demands, I had cut back my dental practice to one day a week. I was devoting twenty-six days a month to answering letters and calls and to seeing one or two mercury-toxic patients per day.

Then came the supreme blow. Although I had been

booked eighteen months in advance, my lecture schedule vaporized.

I had lectured at most of the major national dental meetings, including the national ADA program. I had spent 60 to 100 days a year lecturing to dental groups in the United States, Canada, Mexico, and Europe. My ego was fed by comments like, "That's the first time I sat through an all-day lecture without falling asleep." "You really give us things we can go home and use." "I've never felt so good as since I adopted your program." I was convinced that teaching was my best suit. Then organized dentistry sent out the edict: If you have Huggins on your program, no continuing education credit will be given to the doctors in attendance for the entire program. I was dead in the water.

During this period, there was another fire smoldering within me, one of discontent that was bred from observations of terminal diseases that were "spontaneously" going into remission. Moreover, this spontaneous remission occurred consistently on the fourth or fifth day of treatment. It was remarkable that spontaneity was so predictable.

The academic world asked for controlled studies beyond the scope of private practice. No one seemed to care about recovered patients. Those patients were only "anecdotes," which is a slur word scientists use to refer to human studies that therefore are of little or no value. I didn't have a doctorate, so I was of little or no value either. I felt that academics suffered from paralysis through analysis. They wanted us to re-place amalgam in the recovered patients and duplicate the disease again. I mentioned this to some of the patients. The patients all had the same instructions for me to give the scientific community—they could go to a very warm place. I then vowed that I would make my life's prime objective the exposure of mercury's destructive potential.

After eleven years of ignoring the issue, Joyce Reese, Ph.D., of the NIDR called me in early 1984. The NIDR and the ADA were cosponsoring a conference called the "Workshop on Biocompatibility of Dental Materials" to determine if mercury was a topic worthy of investigation. This meeting turned out to be a result of investigative reporter Tom Bearden's visits to NIDR and ADA, in which he questioned why they were not studying the issue, for his Emmy award-winning series on mercury toxicity. They had lied to him, stating that both organizations were actively investigating the topic. An on-site visit to each organization proved that nothing of the sort was happening. Because of Bearden's questioning, these organizations finally set up a workshop to "investigate."

My thinking had to be direct and organized at the NIDR workshop. I was repeatedly requested to present only patient observations—no scientific studies were acceptable. Dr. Reese, the program chairwoman for the workshop, was very persistent in assuring me that it was the job of the Ph.D.s at the NIDR to determine research maneuvers, not mine. She indicated that my clinical observations were of unique special value. That was an attitude I had never heard from the academic world. I should have known better. I was about to be suckered into my favorite topic, "Look what can be done for people!" I figured it would be best if my clinical observations were limited to chemistries. That's probably what Dr. Reese meant. If I spoke about patients, the term anecdote would surface again, and the Amalgam War would grow cold for another generation.

I began to think of the bottom line. It is a popular buzzword today, and it applies to many more things than accounting. What was my bottom line? To make people aware of the dangers of mercury. What would I have to do to plant that idea? I had given three-day seminars on the subject of mercury alone. Here I would have only forty-five minutes.

I had better be organized (not my strong suit, unfortunately). Then a thought came to mind that became the outline for the presentation: In order for mercury to be a problem, it would have to come out of the filling; form a compound that is toxic; and form a sufficient quantity of this compound to produce disease. Also, remission of symptoms upon amalgam removal would have to be demonstrated.

Having stated the problem, I would have to explain how to diagnose and treat the mercury-toxic patient. But first I had to break down the inertia of the ages and the ingrained assumption that mercury was "tightly bound in an intermetallic compound."

I left for Chicago somewhat apprehensively, bolstered by encouraging words from colleagues and friends, but knowing what the outcome could be. I sat through the first day's presentations, actively ignored by the majority of those in attendance. Few wanted to admit they knew me; fewer yet wanted to be seen talking to me. I listened to the questions asked of the other clinicians by the audience. All seemed to be professionals, and certainly nothing for me to be concerned about. The clinicians for that day seemed to be presenting good information, but with weak conclusions. But after all, this was the academic world, and their jobs would depend upon their not rocking the boat.

When my time came to speak, my opening comments were light and humorous, but no one laughed. No one even cracked a smile. To call them a "hostile audience" would be an understatement. I concluded my presentation; then the question-and-answer session began. The first hangman didn't really want to ask a question; he wanted to disprove a statement I had made. The second wanted only to dress me down in public and vent his anger against me. He never got around to asking a question. The third accused me of interfering with his doctor-patient relationship with a patient I had never seen, never spoken with, and never corresponded with. Again, I was not asked a question. The fourth demanded that I describe all of my "entrepreneurial interests" and financial affairs. And from there the "questions" got worse.

Knowing that my position would be precarious—as the only one of twelve speakers advocating abolition of amalgam—the petite Dr. Reese had jokingly promised to be my bodyguard throughout the proceedings. Where was she when the stones were being thrown? She was sitting with the ADA. Her job was finished, and I was on the chopping block.

It would have been worth all the insults and criticisms had the recommendation of the workshop been to discontinue the use of amalgam until further studies could prove its safety. But the spokespeople did no such thing. Their recommendations boiled down to meaning that no action would be taken because no scientific documentation had been presented to show problems. These conclusions were seen in typed form three hours *before* I presented my material.

The next day, Michael Ziff, D.D.S., a dentist from Florida, was given permission to make a statement. Obviously, he was one of the few who would stick his neck out, and he has done so on numerous occasions since that time. Dr. Ziff gave a speech for the workshop record that included the following statement:

> Advocates of dental mercury amalgam fillings claim that the safety of those fillings has been scientifically proven and documented numerous times and that it has been continuously reaffirmed over the 150 years of its use.

He then proceeded to relate that in September 1981, upon my recommendation, he investigated whether or not mercury could constitute a potential health hazard. He said he first turned to the oral pathology and dental materials textbooks. A chapter by R.W. Phillips in Skinner's *Science of Dental Materials* stated that dental amalgam should not be placed in contact with gold restorations in the oral cavity. In *A Textbook of Oral Pathology* by Schafer, Hines, and Levy he found this statement: "A toxic reaction from absorption of mercury in dental amalgam has been reported on a number of occasions."

Shocked by these findings, he said he next turned to pathology, physiology, pharmacology, chemistry, and other textbooks, and was further alarmed after learning the effects of mercury and its compounds on the human body.

He wrote to the ADA and requested the actual *primary* research establishing the safety of mercury amalgams in patients. The ADA sent one secondary research article (this means that it only quotes the primary article, which is based on actual research) and a form letter stating the ADA position. On it were listed eight references: one was the secondary article; one was a U.S. Government statistical report on dentists; two were primary research papers indicating that mercury is released from amalgams; and four were primary research papers based on urine mercury measurements. The ADA now acknowledges that urine mercury measurements do not correlate to the toxic effects of mercury.

Dr. Ziff then called the ADA and specifically requested the primary research establishing the safety of mercury amalgams in patients. He was told that none was available, and was referred to the NIDR. He then presented the same request to that organization, and was told that there was plenty of research available investigating potential risk to dentists from the use of mercury, but there was none available relating to patient risk, because K.O. Frykholm had proved in 1957 that dental mercury did not present a risk to patients. Frykholm utilized experimental techniques and equipment, including urine mercury measurements, now known to be inadequate.

Dr. Ziff concluded:

> I then turned to the research literature myself. I have now accumulated, read, and documented over 600 references on mercury and dental amalgam. I am absolutely convinced that the use of mercury amalgam in dentistry does constitute a potential health risk to patients.

Dr. Ziff's words were heard without comment.

One member of the audience thanked me for "stepping into the lion's den." This was after the workshop was over and when no one else was around. It sounded nice, but somehow it didn't ease the pain of knowing that nothing would be done. How many more lives would have to be ruined before they capitulated?

I returned to Colorado, temporarily down emotionally, but still determined. After much soul-searching, I decided to write this book to say what needed to be said to you—the public—regardless of the outcome.

# 5

## Dental Materials— The Good, the Bad, and the Ugly

D ental material is a science in itself. We now have well over 1,000 different metallic alloys to choose from. Metals are used in fillings, crowns, partial dentures, orthodontics, and implants. Each company has its own formula for each item, with slight variations to avoid patent infringements.

As people accept the fact that mercury is a poison, the natural question is, "What can be used to fill my teeth?" Boy, does that open up a new subject. During my master's program, one project I was given was to test the immune reactivity of human serum to mercury. The results showed that around 90 percent of the test population was immunoreactive. Next I tested copper, which is highly reactive, even more so than mercury. Finally, I tested all five components of amalgam.

Eventually I set up a laboratory to test all dental materials. Today over 750 materials are tested daily for physicians and dentists all over the world. I have found that no dental material is safe for everyone. Even some of the "safe" plastics react in over 50 percent of the population.

In this chapter, I will examine a few of our options, including gold, amalgam, composites, cast glass, nickel, bases, root canals, and even the effect of cleaning teeth.

## GOLD (THE GOOD)

All that glitters in your mouth may not be gold. Gold is relatively soft, and in its pure state is probably not durable enough for long-term wear. In past years, other metals have been added not only to harden the gold, but also to reduce the cost. Platinum and palladium have been used to harden the metal; now iridium, indium, gallium, silver, and copper are found in gold. Some "golds"actually contain less than 10 percent gold.

Remember that electrical currents in the mouth are implicated in the discharge of materials from fillings, and that contact between any two metals—in your mouth, just as in a battery—generates electrical current. The fewer the metals, the less complex the battery, and the less electrical current it is likely to create. So the higher the percentage of gold, the better the gold may be for you biochemically. Biocompatibility testing helped me discover that even gold is not safe for everyone, however. In testing over 3,500 patients, I found that about 9 percent have an immune system reactivity to gold. Also, many golds contain copper to restore the color lost when white hardeners such as platinum or palladium are added. Copper reacts adversely with over 90 percent of our populace.

No wonder I have problems finding acceptable dental materials. Manufacturers focus on mechanical strength—

not biocompatibility. Yet with such high possible percentages of immune reactivity from all dental materials, we cannot afford to guess. Our immune systems are too precious and are already battered by exposure to pollution and preservatives. I do blood compatibility tests on all of my patients to determine acceptability before placing any dental material.

Combinations of metal alloys create even more problems. Frequently, badly broken teeth are "built up" with amalgam to furnish a foundation for a crown to sit on. Placing gold over amalgam stimulates mercury deposition into the tissues surrounding the tooth's root.

## AMALGAM (THE BAD)

The lay person tends to think of silver fillings as containing primarily silver, gold crowns as being nearly all gold, and porcelain crowns as being made out of ceramic, whatever that is. For ease of communication, this terminology has stood the test of time. After all, who cares that a silver filling has tin, copper, zinc, and mercury in it? And it really *wouldn't* matter if these materials stayed put in the fillings. But they don't. As we have seen, these metals electrochemically slough off, and become part of your body's biochemistry. Those that are poisonous create toxic reactions in your body.

As if conventional amalgams were not bad enough, there is now the very popular high-copper amalgam. Chemically, the high-copper amalgams emit mercury *fifty times faster* than conventional amalgams. Clinically, when a person becomes ill due to high-copper amalgam, it is extremely difficult to correct his or her disturbances. High-copper amalgams should be entirely avoided even if you are not personally concerned about mercury toxicity. Ask your dentist what type of amalgam material he or she uses. Don't allow *anyone* to place high-copper amalgam in your mouth or the mouths of your family members. Of all the metallic dental materials, high-copper amalgam is probably the most deadly.

## COMPOSITES (GOOD AND BAD)

What can be used in place of amalgam? Is anything available that is comparable in cost and durability? The University of Colorado School of Dentistry studied the longevity of amalgam fillings and came up with this statement: "The half-life of amalgam is four years." This means that if 100 amalgams were placed today, 50 would still be in the mouth four years from now; 25 would still be in service eight years from now; 12 to 13 would still be there in twelve years, and about 6 would still be left in twenty years.

Composites, filling materials made out of ground glass powder mixed with a plastic binder, require more time to place than amalgam, so they can be expected to cost perhaps ten to twenty dollars more. There is no data on their life span comparable to the University of Colorado study, but many have been known to pass the five- and ten-year marks. Manufacturers are improving the mechanics of composites each year.

Composites come in two basic forms, light cure and chemical cure. With the light-cured materials, the material is placed into the tooth in a plastic form. A special light is then concentrated on the material that causes it to harden in place. Chemically cured fillings consist of two pastes. When they are mixed together, a chemical reaction is set up that hardens the material.

Some people who have allergies can tolerate the light cure better than the chemical cure because the latter takes longer to cure. Composite materials seem to be suitable for about 50 percent of the patients I see. The other 50 percent experience immune reactivity. Although this is a step in the right direction, there are still many immunoreactive chemicals in these fillings. That 50-50 chance is why I do serum compatibility testing on each and every patient.

Are composites safe? In a study of 7,000 ambulatory dental patients representing a wide distribution of people ages 10 to 80 from all geographic areas including the United States, Europe, Australia, New Zealand, and Canada, 64 percent reacted to over 50 percent of the composites. In fact, one of the most popular "plastic" fillings shows immune reactivity in over 90 percent of the population.

## NICKEL (THE UGLY)

Despite its known allergenic properties, carcinogenicity, and toxicity, nickel has wormed its way into the biggest slice of the casting material market today. In some parts of the country, nickel is used in over 90 percent of the crowns made. Overall use is around 80 percent. Many patients I see thought they were getting gold crowns. They weren't.

Nickel is used in place of gold to make crowns for badly broken-down teeth when cost is a factor. Its major use is as a base onto which porcelain is fired. This is how porcelain crowns or caps are made. Even though nickel is used in many removable bridges, the metal appears to be more detrimental in the form used for crowns. Most of the adverse reactions to nickel are similar to those of mercury toxicity. Neurological disturbances, emotional upsets, and blood problems (like leukemia) can be initiated by nickel crowns.

Most removable bridges, called partial dentures, are made of nickel. When I used to place nickel partials in patients, I had to baby-sit them for the first two weeks of "adjustment." The typical patient salivated more and felt

like he had a horseshoe in his mouth. But with persist-
ence, understanding, and carefully placed guilt trips, I
was successful in helping patients wear those toxic appliances.

However, during my last two years of active wet-fin-
ger dentistry, I placed only gold partials. The cost was
about $150 more because the lesser strength and greater
weight per volume of gold caused the partials to be
thicker and heavier than conventional nickel partials.
Despite this extra thickness and weight, people got along
with them fine. They did not notice the bulkiness because
the metal was not toxic. Gold can be cast with amazing
accuracy, so the fits were terrific. The patient felt fine, had
no excessive salivation, and had no periodic removal
while becoming adjusted. I wonder . . . does the body
know that nickel is highly toxic and gold is not?

One thing I am beginning to note about nickel and
other nongold metals is that they frequently create negative electrical current in the mouth. Nickel and a palla-
dium-silver-tin metal we have seen a lot lately in crowns
have both registered negative current in some very ill
patients. So it saves you thirty or forty dollars per crown.
Is it worth it? Ask the epileptic, the patient with MS, or the
person with leukemia who is counting his last days. What
a price to pay for economy!

If you as a patient choose nickel, I have no objection. I
just don't want a dentist or anyone else making that kind
of decision about your health without consulting you or
giving you a choice.

Nickel has been used in children for several decades in
the form of metallic preformed crowns on badly decayed
baby teeth. They are called chrome crowns, but are really
nickel-containing stainless steel crowns. Many of these
emit negative electrical current. They set up an electrical
relationship with other metals, like amalgam, and create

a "battery" in the mouth that emits mercury and the other metals.

Tin-grin orthodontic patients are showing off nickel, not tin. The amount of electrical current generated by braces is generally several times higher than that created by amalgam fillings. The current can be either positive or negative. I have seen positive current in one arch and negative in the other. All this additional electrical current, combined with that from amalgam, can create many types of metal compounds that jump into your saliva, forming a real corrosion soup that you swallow.

Allergists have told me that when they have a slightly allergic patient who is going to get braces, they brace themselves. They know that the allergies are going to get worse. Most of these doctors are not aware of this mechanism or they would have complained years ago. With the increase in electrical activity, all chemical reactions proceed faster. This includes mercury coming out of the fillings, disrupting white blood cell metabolism and stimulating allergic reactions. Some of the worst reactions I have seen occurred when the patients had combinations of nickel, gold, and amalgam, for instance when amalgam and gold restoration were present under orthodontic bands.

## CAST GLASS (SNEAKY)

There is now a new generation of cast glass crowns and inlays coming on the market. From the standpoint of bio-compatibility, they contain more than 25 percent aluminum, in the form of aluminum oxide. This figure may be as high as 45 percent in some porcelains. Just as in the case of mercury in amalgam, dentists have been led to believe that all components are tightly bound and safe. However,

I recommend that you have your immune system tested before allowing your dentist to place cast glass in your mouth. Over 80 percent of dental patients suffer a drop in immune protection when exposed to aluminum.

## BASES (SO-SO, BUT NECESSARY)

Metals like gold, nickel, and amalgam conduct heat and cold faster than tooth enamel. This is one reason why teeth are sensitive to temperature changes after a new filling is placed. Another reason is negative electrical current generated by high-copper amalgams. Electricity can make teeth supersensitive for years. In order to reduce the thermal shock from items like coffee and ice cream, a dentist will frequently place a coat of insulation, called a base, over the pulp chamber where the nerve lives. This has always been considered a very helpful thing to do for the patient's benefit. Now I am finding that Dycal, the most often used base material, gives many people a reaction similar to that caused by mercury. I have no idea why this is true, but enough patients have had to have their dentistry redone because of these reactions to make me hesitant to use or recommend it. The manufacturer is highly resistant to discussing the product.

What is the best base? The one that is biocompatible for you. I don't guess anymore. I do the blood test to find out which one is least reactive to your immune system.

## ROOT CANALS (BAD *AND* UGLY)

A root canal is a tooth that has had the nerve removed and replaced with a sterile material, a heavy wax or paste. This is usually done because a tooth has died. Teeth may die due to trauma (such as a blow or fall in which the tooth is hit and the nerve is killed), or a break in a tooth that exposes the nerve, or decay that reaches the nerve and infects it with bacteria. The most common sign of the need for a root canal is when a tooth causes pain that will not go away. When hot things (like coffee) touch a tooth and cause such pain that you go through the ceiling, this is usually a sign of a dead tooth. Another indicator is a dental x-ray that reveals an area at the root tip where the bone has been dissolved by infection. Also, there may be pus around the tooth.

Root canal filling, in which the space formerly occupied by a dental nerve is filled, can be done in two ways. Usually a hole is cut from the top of the tooth into the nerve chamber, and the chamber is filled through that hole. Another method is used when the abscess is farther advanced. This involves cutting through the bone at the root end, cleaning out all the infected material there, sealing the root tip, and sewing the area together. Bone is supposed to fill in the defect. Amalgam is then usually used to seal the pulp chamber at the root tip.

Retrograde filling is the term applied to this type of root canal sealing process. With a retrograde filling, mercury has direct access to the body fluids and can cause problems similar to those created by amalgam in the mouth. The only difference is that fillings in the mouth are much easier to replace.

About five years ago I was introduced to the hazards of root canals. I had a patient who responded dramatically upon the removal of five of them. A few more patients responded in equally dramatic fashion, and that stimulated an investigation. I have found nothing more vicious than the reactions people have to root canals. This is not a new discovery, either. Weston Price, D.D.S., M.S., director of research for the ADA for fourteen years, published many articles in the 1920s telling of the dangers of root-filled teeth. Just try to find those materials now. Reactions don't hit people the day they are placed, unless their immune systems are in tip-top condition. In that case, the recently filled root canal tooth will grow pus and create abundant pain—just the opposite of what dentists are taught in school.


## THE EFFECT OF CLEANING TEETH

The long-accepted practice of cleaning teeth and polishing amalgam fillings can have an adverse effect as well as a good one. Cleaning the teeth presents no problems at all where there is no amalgam present. But polishing with pumice (done after the plaque and calculus or tartar are removed) removes a layer of corrosion from amalgams. This increases the amount of mercury vapor coming off the fillings into your body.

I'm not saying that you shouldn't have your teeth cleaned, just that if you are reactive to mercury, you should have your amalgams removed first. More and more of my patients are telling me that they have increased symptoms after having their teeth cleaned. It is certainly easy to understand why.

What am I doing about these dental materials? I test every mercury-toxic patient before amalgam removal to assure patients and myself that I am using state-of-the-art methods of determining biocompatibility, to combat the effects of state-of-the-art high-copper amalgams.

Progress is being made, however. November 5–10, 1988, I cosponsored with the University of Colorado the International Conference on Biocompatibility of Materials (ICBM). It was attended by researchers, physicians, and dentists from thirteen nations. At the end of the conference, the speakers voted unanimously to sign the following declaration:

Based on the known toxic potentials of mercury and its documented release from dental amalgams, usage of mercury-containing amalgam increases the health risk of the patients, the dentists, and the personnel.

This statement is a landmark conclusion for dentistry. It demonstrates the key concept that is the focus of this book: The individual biocompatibility of a material should be fully evaluated before it is placed within the patient.

The success of the conference will ultimately be measured by how long it takes to eliminate toxic substances from the practice of dentistry. Until then, I continue to test patients to find the least offensive materials for their individual immune systems.

# 6
# Diagnosing
# Mercury Toxicity

One of the most often asked questions, as you might guess, is, "How do I find out if I am mercury toxic?" It sounds logical that a blood or urine test for the presence of mercury would answer that question. However, biochemistry does not always take the logical routes we would like it to. Over the years, it has become evident to me that it is not the *presence* of mercury that counts, but a person's *reactivity* to mercury. True, if no mercury is present, there can be no reaction. But the problem is that it takes very little mercury to react in people who are sensitive.

Sensitivity varies for all people. In this chapter, I will expand on prior discussion of the new, positive test for mercury toxicity, the urine porphyrin test, and I will show you a series of tests that I use in diagnosis and in formulating a treatment program.

## COULD YOU HAVE MERCURY TOXICITY?

What if mercury is present? What does it mean? The bloodstream is the primary avenue for mercury to enter and exit the body. But according to James Woods, Ph.D., of the University of Washington, if an atom of mercury enters the bloodstream, another atom will exit six one-millionths of a second later. Barring sudden extreme exposures, then, the bloodstream levels of mercury tend to be rather constant.

Recent dental journal articles by Drs. C.W. Svare and D.D. Gay show that there is a relationship between blood levels of mercury and the number of silver-mercury fillings present in the mouth. David Eggleston, D.D.S., of California and Magnus Nylander, D.D.S., Ph.D., of Karolinska Institute in Stockholm, Sweden, have researched and published articles showing that at autopsy, people's brain levels of mercury corresponded with the number of silver fillings in their mouths.

Are you mercury toxic? Can your mercury level be tested? These are simple questions, but the answers are complicated. Mercury attacks many systems in the body. If it attacked just one, like the polio and measles viruses do, it would be quite easy to identify. The diagnosis of mercury toxicity must instead be based on the number of changes that occur in the body and the degree of these changes. For example, white blood cells usually increase as a response to the introduction of amalgam. If these cells go up from a 5,000 count (indicating 5,000 white blood cells per cubic millimeter of blood) to a 7,000 count, it is not especially notable. If the count goes from 5,000 to 50,000, which is quite notable, we may be talking about leukemia. The white blood cell count bears much more weight in diagnosis at 50,000 than 7,000.

Patients usually think in terms of symptoms, but doctors are apt to look for measurable parameters. There are a number of standard medical tests that can help your doctor to determine: 1) where your body was damaged; 2) to what extent it was damaged; and 3) what challenge condition precipitated the damage.

The following are considered chemical indicators or early warning signs of mercury toxicity:

- A white blood cell count above 7,500 or below 4,500.

- Hematocrit above 50 percent or below 40 percent (this is the percentage by volume of packed red blood cells in a sample of blood after it has been spun in a centrifuge).

- A lymphocyte count above 2,800 or below 1,800 (lymphocytes are a type of white blood cells that function in the development of immunity).

- A blood protein level above 7.5 grams per 100 milliliters of serum (7.5 g percent ml).

- A blood triglyceride level above 150 mg percent ml.

- A blood urea nitrogen (BUN) level above 18 or below 12 percent.

- A level of nickel in the hair above 1.5 parts per million (ppm).

- A hair mercury level above 1.5 ppm or below 0.4 ppm.

- A hair aluminum level above 15 ppm.

- A hair manganese level below 0.3 ppm.

- Immune reactions to aluminum, nickel, mercury, copper, or gold.

- Oxyhemoglobin below 55 percent saturation (oxyhemoglobin is the oxygen-carrying element in the blood; saturation refers to the percentage of oxygen in it).

- Carboxyhemoglobin above 2.5 percent saturation (carboxyhemoglobin is a compound formed in the blood when inhaled carbon monoxide combines with hemoglobin).

- T-lymphocytes (a subset of the lymphocyte family) that have been inactivated by mercury. The lymphocyte is the primary white blood cell involved in immune defense reactions in the body. Its chief function is to manufacture immunoglobulins, one of the major fighters in the immune system. When these cells are attacked, the count goes down to below 2,000 per cubic millimeter (the normal range is 2,200 to 2,400).

- DNA analysis (a measurement of the content of genetic material within a cell) that reveals mercury-induced malignancies. Within the lymphocyte is DNA, which contains your personal genetic code. Mercury can cause two DNA chains to combine, doubling the number of chromosomes present (from forty-eight to ninety-six). By definition, this is malignancy.

Other factors that indicate special scrutiny may be warranted are:

- The presence of root canal-treated teeth.
- Telltale combinations of symptoms. For instance, I might see a patient with multiple sclerosis and a low body temperature, or someone with chronic fatigue syndrome and brainfog and short-term memory loss.
- The presence of both amalgam and gold.
- Magnitude of polarity of electrical current. Electricity indicates the speed of chemical reactions on the surface of a filling. The higher the magnitude, the greater the speed. Also, negative electric current is worse than positive. It fosters faster conversion of mercury into methyl mercury.

These are just some signs of potential mercury toxicity. The intensity and direction of each reaction must also be considered. For instance, a glucose level that goes from 90 to 190 milligrams per 100 milliliters of blood indicates the onset of diabetes, so clearly this is motion in the wrong direction. Conversely, if blood sugar went from 190 to 90 milligrams per 100 milliliters, it would be heading in the right direction. Obviously, the diagnosis of mercury toxicity is a professional judgment call. And since each reaction has the potential to affect several others, it becomes increasingly important to rely upon professional judgment rather than a single test result.

However, as mentioned in Chapter 1, there is one single test that does show great promise, the urine porphyrin test. Porphyrins are chemicals that form the compound adenosine triphosphate (ATP), which provides the energy for all the cells in the body. Interference with the process that turns porphyrins into ATP is proof of serious metabolic disturbance. Recently it has been shown that mercury inhibits the action of an enzyme that is critical to the series of events leading to ATP production. Not only that, but mercury creates a distinctive pattern of interference that differentiates it from other heavy metals.

From the lay standpoint, how would you suspect that you are affected by mercury? Probably one of the simplest ways is to look at the list of symptoms and diseases that we have seen respond most often to amalgam removal, as discussed in Chapter 3.

Should everyone just run right out and have all of his or her fillings removed? That's not wise. First of all, not everyone responds to an amalgam by developing dreaded disease. I would certainly recommend never having another amalgam placed, but not everyone needs to have his or her amalgams removed. Then who *does* need amalgam removal? Obviously people with nonresponsive diseases, especially the diseases discussed in this book. If you suffer from annoying symptoms that you wish would go away so you could enjoy a more pleasant life, you may wish to consider it. Remember, *unexplained* is the key word with mercury toxicity. If that is how your doctor classifies your symptoms, the odds are that some type of toxicity may be involved. If your decision is to get rid of amalgam, the following course of action is what I have found most beneficial for your guidance.

Knowing the state of your health and body chemistry prior to amalgam removal will enable your doctor to use all biochemical parameters needed before beginning amalgam removal. In other words, a doctor who has read your blood chemistry reports knows your excesses and deficiencies, and can alter these by recommending modifications in your diet and/or the addition or subtraction of nutritional supplements. If proper nutrition and supplementation are initiated prior to amalgam removal, there is a greater chance of success. It will also enable him or her to guide your progress through follow-up testing after the procedure. Sometimes several subtle changes are all that are needed to help guide a patient toward good health.

## DIAGNOSTIC TESTING PROCEDURES

I have a standard starting point, or minimum number of tests, that gives me an adequate basis from which a treatment plan can be established. In addition to the urine porphyrin test, these tests include:

- A blood serum profile.
- A hair analysis for presence of toxic metals.
- A complete blood count (CBC) with differential and platelet count.

- Urinary mercury excretion.
- Electrical current.
- A health questionnaire.

In the mercury-toxic patient, I look at the specific elements of body chemistry that relate directly to mercury toxicity. This does not imply that the other aspects of body chemistry are not important. They are just not addressed at the initial appointment.

Not all of the potential changes in body chemistry occur in every mercury-toxic patient. Neither is toxicity related specifically to how many areas are affected. Overall, if you were to evaluate 100 patients, you would find that greater disease problems are apt to be associated with greater chemical disturbances. But on an individual basis, that doesn't always hold true.

One common denominator that you may notice cropping up again and again is mercury's attraction to the sulfur-containing compounds in the body. This information is very helpful in explaining some reactions, like a lack of energy in people whose blood test results look great.

The following are the testing procedures that I use as a guide in treating the mercury-toxic patient.

### Urine Porphyrin Test

The urine porphyrin test is perhaps the best indicator of heavy metal toxicity. According to research by Dr. James Woods at the University of Washington, mercury toxicity appears to leave a specific fingerprint in the excretion of a chemical called porphyrin. From the practical standpoint, however, no one has only mercury in his or her mouth. Most of my patients have amalgam, but amalgam is a combination of mercury, copper, tin, zinc, and silver.

Many have root canals and cavitations (holes in the bone where an old extraction site has not completely healed) as well.

I have found that all of these, and possibly a few other heavy metals as well, cause an increase in the excretion of porphyrins. Porphyrins are chemicals that the body manufactures for the purpose of transporting energy for use by every cell in the body. Gasoline is a good fuel, and so is kerosene, but for different types of engines. Similarly, the prophyrins turn into more than one product, depending on the body's requirements.

One key product of porphyrins is hemoglobin, perhaps the best known energy unit in the body. Hemoglobin's primary function is to transport oxygen from the lungs to all body tissues. Through a series of chemical maneuvers, porphyrin turns into a molecule called *heme*, which can combine with another chemical, called *globin*, to become the familiar hemoglobin molecule.

Heme is also the basis for the conversion of the carbohydrates, proteins, and fats we eat into energy that the cells can use. This happens by means of a process called cellular respiration, in which a series of enzymatic reactions take place within the mitochondria (tiny subunits within cells) that release carbon and hydrogen from the foods we eat. As these atoms are plucked off our foods, energy is released. This energy is captured, so to speak, in a process in which a chemical known as adenosine diphosphate (ADP) is converted into adenosine triphosphate (ATP). ATP is the storage unit that provides fuel for all life processes within the body. Heme—made from porphyrin—is a factor primary in this capture and conversion process.

However, when mercury, copper, or substances within root-canaled teeth are released within the body, they can inactivate the enzymes that help to form heme from porphyrin, or they can prevent heme from assisting in the energy-capturing process that converts ADP into ATP. When this happens, heme formation backs up and porphyrins spill over from the blood into the urine. Your energy is literally flushed down the toilet as porphyrins in your urine. No wonder you have chronic fatigue!

Originally, I had thought that the porphyrin test would be a specific test for mercury, but I have found that it can tell about many other toxicities as well. The effects of braces, root canals, chrome crowns, the popular and inexpensive nickel crowns (frequently covered with porcelain), and amalgam fillings can all be monitored. If the removal of any of these materials leads to a significant reduction in the amount of porphyrins being excreted in the urine, it becomes obvious that those materials were interfering with energy production. Monitoring the excretion of porphyrins in urine is a good way to measure the success of treatment.

## Blood Serum Profile

The blood has two components, cells and serum. The serum is the fluid portion, from which the cells have been removed. In a blood serum profile, a long series of tests determines the amounts of certain chemicals—such as glucose, cholesterol, and triglycerides—present in the blood. These are the chemicals that keep our bodies running.

*Glucose, cholesterol, and triglycerides.* The first thing I look for in blood serum chemistry is the relationship between glucose, cholesterol, and triglycerides. If a person is eating more carbohydrate than would be found in his or her ancestral diet—the combination of foods that your genetic ancestors have eaten for the last one to two thousand years—most often the levels of all three of these substances will be elevated. If that is the case, I look to nutritional factors. On the other hand, if mercury is offending the chemistry, I may see a slight elevation of glucose (blood sugar) and a suppression of cholesterol, while the triglycerides skyrocket.

The level of glucose in the blood is regulated by the hormone insulin, which is manufactured by the pancreas. The process of synthesizing insulin requires the formation of sulfur-based bonds between two chains of molecules. Mercury, by interfering with sulfur binding sites, can inhibit the production of insulin; an insufficient level of insulin can then cause the glucose level to elevate. If your insulin is particularly susceptible to interference from mercury, your glucose levels can get high enough for you to be considered diabetic. Chromium, manganese, vitamin C, and diet play a big role in diabetes, so mercury is not the major factor. But it can be a contributing factor that doesn't need to be there, and one that can complicate getting well.

Cholesterol is a constituent in all cell membranes and is very important in the construction of hormones. Advertising has focused on the negative side of cholesterol, without letting us in on the fact that it is *essential* for life. In fact, cholesterol is so important that the body manufactures the majority of it from the non-cholesterol-containing foods we eat. There is a chemical pathway in the body's metabolism that is called the Krebs citric acid cycle. One of the cycle's byproducts is a substance called succinic acid, which is a building block for cholesterol. Mercury can interfere with the production of succinic acid, which in turn reduces the total amount of cholesterol that can be manufactured.

Blood cholesterol can be lowered by excess exercise, to a point below what the dietary factors of sugar, alcohol, and caffeine would predict. Interference from mercury can lower this level even more, so for the causes of a really low cholesterol level—one so low that it retards hormonal development—we must explore beyond nutrition. Mercury can be a culprit, too. An abnormally low cholesterol level can lead to the production of less thyroid hormone, estrogen, testosterone, and probably other potential hormonal disturbances.

The telltale combination of high glucose and low cholesterol is, as "science" would say, "suggestive" of a problem, but since it does not occur 100 percent of the time, it cannot be considered a positive diagnosis. An individual genetic pattern may also be involved, which would explain why not all people with high glucose and low cholesterol are reactive. Since cholesterol is the basis for the adrenocortical hormones (like estrogen and testosterone), this interrelationship could suggest the arenas of some of the hormonal interferences observed in mercury-toxic patients. The glucose-cholesterol movement alone might suggest a relationship between mercury and diabetes. Amalgam removal has even resulted in a lowering of some diabetics' insulin requirements. For patients who do not take insulin, amalgam removal has helped to bring down elevated glucose levels significantly.

A person's triglyceride level is a measurement of fats in the blood. Triglycerides are a thick, gummy substance that causes the heart to push harder to keep the blood flowing. Elevated triglyceride levels can be associated with high blood pressure. A variety of things affect triglycerides. Excess carbohydrate intake elevates triglycerides faster than sugar intake affects glucose, for example. I have seen cases in which glucose and cholesterol are in the proper range while the triglyceride level is elevated 100 to 300 points. This is quite a movement, since the desired range is 100 micrograms or less per 100 milliliters of blood. A difference of several hundred percent is quite significant when it concerns something that tends to make the blood serum thick. This is often due to the body's response to the presence of mercury. In some of these cases, the triglyceride level later dropped 200 points within three days after amalgam removal. In other cases, emotional stress will cause several hundred points of elevation. This is where a doctor has to balance nutrition against emotional stress against mercury in making a diagnostic judgment. When mercury is causing a problem with triglycerides, though, changes are dramatic and fast following proper amalgam removal and replacement with compatible substances.

*Blood serum proteins.* Blood serum proteins are the next area of interest, and yield more specific diagnoses. There are two basic serum proteins: albumin and globulin. They are both participants in our immune system. Because of their interrelationships, I consider the white blood cells and serum proteins together when evaluating a patient's immune defense system.

Many people have heard the term gamma globulin, or have even had a gamma globulin shot to bolster their immune system. When mercury enters the bloodstream, the immune system reacts against this foreign material by increasing the amount of globulin. How does mercury get into the bloodstream? As mercury vapor comes off of dental fillings, it can be inhaled, and it can pass from the lungs directly into the bloodstream. Further, if the vapor mixes with food during chewing, it can be swallowed, enter the digestive tract, and be absorbed into the bloodstream. Either way, when mercury gets into the bloodstream, the immune system is going to react.

Mercury in vapor form is highly reactive chemically, and starts looking for those delicious sulfur bonds. Albumin has some of these tasty sulfurs, so it becomes a favorite dining place for mercury. Mercury grabs hold. When mercury grabs one of these sulfur binding sites, it holds on with a death grip. Then globulin comes along. Globulin's job description is to destroy strangers in the blood. A mercury-albumin compound will certainly look like a stranger. How does the body deal with it? The immune system chooses to cover the mercury compound with a coat of globulin. With a covering of globulin, the compound becomes transparent, or invisible to the immune system. The immune system no longer includes that compound in its census of strangers.

Mercury is still floating around in the blood, even though it is bound to albumin and coated with globulin. A blood test may show a slightly elevated globulin level. As more mercury seeps into the blood, more coatings appear, and the globulin level goes up a little more. This increase is slow, like a cat creeping up on a bird. Since most people have amalgam in their mouths, this creeping up of the globulin level is common, therefore classified as a normal occurrence, and little attention is paid to it.

Since part of the treatment of the mercury-toxic patient is to remove this globulin (a process called globulin-stripping), the status of the immune system becomes more and more significant. Observations have suggested to me that a patient's ability to respond after amalgam removal is somehow related to the multiple abilities of the immune system. When this idea first began to take form, I looked at total protein levels, albumin levels, globulin levels, and the albumin-to-globulin ratio (A/G ratio). None of these consistently told what I needed to find out. Then I realized that globulin was telling the story, but only if you looked at its relationship to the total amount of protein in the blood. This created a new ratio—the total protein-to-globulin ratio (TP/G). This is determined by dividing the total protein value (the amount of albumin *and* globulin) by the globulin value. For instance, if the total protein is

7.0 grams per 100 milliliters (g percent ml) and the globulin is 2.4 g percent ml, then the TP/G ratio is 2.9/1 (or, for
simplicity's sake, 2.9).

In looking back over patient records, I found that this
ratio holds a key to diagnosis. Patients with ratios around
2.9 to 3.1 responded quickly to treatment. Those with a
ratio below 2.6 responded more slowly, and those below
2.1 were even slower reactors. How can you change the
ratio? I found that vitamin A and a combination of minerals and digestive enzymes will correct it in most people.
Vitamin A seems to be the biggest single factor in speeding
up recovery reactions as shown by this ratio.

Today I check the TP/G ratio early in diagnosis. Ratios
close to 3.0 suggest that I tell the patient to expect a speedy
recovery. Lower ratios suggest that the patient pay close
attention to dietary intake and watch carefully for other
mercury exposures that might hamper progress.


## Hair Analysis

In scrutinizing patient chemistries for evidence of mercury
toxicity, hair analysis is helpful. Hair analysis has been
performed for several decades to determine mineral content
in hair. Minerals found in the hair include calcium, manganese, mercury, zinc, and potassium. Hair analysis involves
doing a chemical washing/stripping of all substances on the
hair, then dissolving the hair in acids. A certain amount of it
(by weight) is dissolved in a known volume of acid. Then,
using a method of chemical analysis called atomic absorption photospectrometry, each mineral is isolated and measured on a parts-per-million (ppm) basis.

There have been many theories as to what the results
of hair analysis do and do not mean. During the years from
1968 to 1983, I saw probably half a million individual

mineral analyses. At that time, I was teaching blood chemistry as a diagnostic tool to determine the relationship between dental decay, gum disease, and nutrition. Hair analysis expanded the parameters of diagnosis.

Hair analysis is a unique analysis. One of the criticisms that has been leveled at it is that it does not reflect what is going on in the blood. Well, this is why it is a unique analysis. It is unique in the things that it shows. Some chemistries mirror those found in the blood; some are the opposite. For example, when hair analysis shows low levels of sodium or potassium, it generally reflects a deficiency in the cells. The levels of sodium or potassium in the blood, meanwhile, may well be *higher* than normal, because the body is trying to get more of the minerals into those deficient cells. In other words, what we see in the blood represents a corrective process for the situation in the cells, not the situation itself. Conversely, high levels of sodium and potassium in the hair analysis are frequently seen in conjunction with low levels in the blood. As heavy metal levels are detected in hair, it is the interpretation of these levels (through correlation with the blood values and other metals) that is the important part, not the level itself. Low nickel levels indicate low exposure, which is not much of a problem. Low mercury levels, on the other hand, may indicate that the body is retaining mercury, and therefore suggests trouble. After treatment, the same low level may indicate lack of exposure and ensuing health.

*The calcium-manganese-mercury triad.* Many of our patients have a condition I call the triad, or a characteristic imbalance of three minerals: calcium, manganese, and mercury. Most often calcium is high, especially in females. High is defined as above 1,100 ppm, and may go up to 5,000 or more in a female. Levels of 2,000 ppm are very high for a male. At the low end of the scale, calcium can appear in the 200 to 300 ppm range.

In a study of thirty women with premenstrual syndrome (PMS), I found that nearly every one had an elevated calcium level, as well as having the general pattern for the mercury-toxic patient in other aspects of body chemistry. Is it possible that such a widespread problem could be caused by amalgams? Remember the interference with hormones that has already been discussed? Add to that the excess calcium levels. It certainly does appear that amalgams could play a role in this common female affliction.

There are different interpretations of the various combinations of imbalances in the triad, but let's start with the worst: high calcium, low manganese, and low mercury. This combination is seen in the most severe cases, and is the toughest to correct. What appears to happen is that mercury combines with a chemical on the cell membrane, the cell's "skin." This mercury-chemical combination has an affinity for calcium. When the mercury and calcium become incorporated in the cell membrane, the membrane's instructions on how to transfer oxygen into the cell and carbon dioxide out of the cell become confused. Because of this confusion, oxygen enters the cells more slowly, and carbon dioxide is released more slowly, resulting in an overall inefficiency of internal cellular metabolism. Clinical observations also suggest that mercury is not excreted as effectively when the calcium levels are high.

Low manganese is a problem because it seems to be a large factor in all the diseases that have been mentioned. In my studies, I have noted that manganese is apt to be the primary mineral deficiency in degenerative diseases. Mercury can be toxic in itself. It can also combine with other substances to form methyl mercury, which is even more toxic. Either form can inhibit the action of manganese. Manganese acts as a key to unlocking the energy in a cell; if mercury interferes, then the cell doesn't function properly. The academic question then becomes: Does mercury interference cause the problem or does lack of manganese action cause the problem?

Paradoxically, a high manganese level produces the same effect as a low one, because as mineral levels go up beyond the optimum ranges, they appear to be in a non-biological (inactive) form. They behave as if they are not reactive. The net result is that this produces the same effect on the body as a low level.

High manganese levels (above 1.0 part per million) are not common. They are seen in roughly 10 percent of the thousands of analyses I have done. Adding a supplement called TransMix to the diet helps to rid the body of the inactive mineral, and then fresh minerals can do their work.

The level of mercury in the hair gives a clue as to how the body may be reacting. A low level indicates a lack of ability to excrete, meaning that toxicity may exist because the body cannot rid itself of mercury quickly enough (retention toxicity). High levels indicate a greater-than-average exposure and simultaneously suggest an increased ability to excrete mercury. I once thought that low levels suggested low exposure, but that does not seem to be the case. Today, low levels suggest that I am going to have difficulty in treating a case. As a result, more attention must be paid to diet, exercise, and other chemistries, like hormone levels.

The bottom line for the effect of the triad can be summed up as an alteration of cell membrane permeability. Each cell has a tendency to absorb or reject surrounding chemicals. When these three minerals get out of balance, the cell membrane can start letting in more toxins, which results in the manufacture of improper products.

*Zinc and potassium.* Establishment of the triad (calcium, manganese, and mercury) gives a starting point for mercury toxicity as far as hair analysis is concerned. Next I look to two other minerals. If a patient is really toxic, I see the triad extend to deficiencies of zinc and potassium. Potassium becomes involved in severe neurological problems like emotional disturbances, epilepsy, and MS.

As a general rule, the more deficient a patient is in zinc and potassium (in that order), the more problems he or she is likely to have. Both are involved in so many chemical reactions in the body that it is difficult to pinpoint why they are so important.

Both zinc and potassium can also be found in the excessively high ranges. And just as in the case of manganese, the excessive amounts seem to be inactive and the symptoms are those of deficiency. This happens perhaps 15 percent of the time, so it is not a widespread problem, but it is becoming more notable all the time. Usually excessive zinc levels are related to eating too much hard cheese. For people with high zinc levels, hard cheese must be severely restricted for three to six months while the zinc level is optimizing.

There are other minerals that can affect the activity of all of these minerals, but they are not common, and they are not typical reactors like these five.

### Complete Blood Count

A complete blood count (CBC) is an action-packed analysis. It is among the least costly tests (ten dollars, more or less, in most areas), yet provides a lot of information for diagnosis and for follow-up. I look first at the white blood cell count. When white cells are elevated or depressed at all, it is important to look at what is called the *differential*. This is a count of white cells that divides them into several families. I am finding that some of the families (monocytes, eosinophils, and basophils) that were thought to be normal for most people do not regularly show up when mercury is not present. These cells can double, triple, or disappear within two or three days (depending on the body's response to amalgam removal), which is dramatic when you consider the trillions of blood cells the body contains.

Overall, this most useful analysis parallels one of my most practical discoveries. Most people who suffer from mercury toxicity are constantly fatigued. They sleep more than eight hours a night and wake up tired. Many have been to a physician for chronic fatigue and have had a blood test done. The red cells and hemoglobin were excellent so they were told to see a psychiatrist because, "It's all in your head."

Well over half of my patients have followed this pattern. They feel insulted by the suggestion that they are using fatigue as a sham to avoid obligation. After seeing this pattern in hundreds of patients, even before I was aware of mercury toxicity, I began to wonder what biochemical explanation could lie behind the syndrome. Dr. Al Belian, who bugs me by dropping new ideas on me every few months, called with an idea that became what I feel is the answer. Remember those sulfur bonds I mentioned in the blood profile section? Dr. Belian told me that hemoglobin has four of these binding sites on each molecule, and that mercury can easily attach to them.

Then I started thinking. What if one mercury atom got onto one sulfur position out of the four possible? Hemoglobin's oxygen-carrying capacity would drop 25 percent. Could a 25-percent drop in oxygen make someone feel fatigued? Couldn't inefficient transport produce the same effect as low hemoglobin? Then I noticed another interesting point. Some of those patients had quite good hemoglobin levels, even higher than high normal. Further, they had a high hematocrit. Hematocrit is a term used to indicate the percentage of blood that is composed of red blood cells. I have noted that when all biochemical and nutritional systems are in balance, the hematocrit is usually 44 to 46 percent. Normal, as seen by hospital laboratories, can extend down to 38 percent. Yet some of my fatigued patients were running as high as 52 to 54 percent. That doesn't make sense. Unless . . . what if the body recognizes that it is not transporting enough oxygen, and it compensates for this deficiency by crowding more red blood cells into the bloodstream? That would produce a high concentration of low-efficiency hemoglobin. The result of this is a good-looking blood chemistry, and a fatigued, "anemic" patient who makes the pilgrimage from doctor to doctor.

Another finding from an entirely different area cropped up about the same time. Dr. Olympio Pinto had recorded on videotape the changes in live red blood cells caused by eating pork, smoking cigarettes, drinking caffeine, and other potentially destructive habits. Of particular interest to me was the profound reaction of a patient one hour after he ate pork. I noted that more than half of his red blood cells were then what are termed "ghosts." Ghosts are red cells that have lost their hemoglobin. (Hemoglobin, in addition to being the carrier of energy-giving oxygen, is also the pigment that makes red blood cells red.) This could explain the sleepiness people get after eating. Most people call it hypoglycemia, but if you consider the ghost cells, it looks as if a lack of oxygen transport is a more logical answer.

Dr. Pinto pointed out that amalgam placement does the same thing to red cells. He also suggested that the act of eating could generate enough mercury vapor to ghost a significant number of red cells. I asked Dr. David Bowerman how, if at least 50 percent of your red cells are nonfunctional, and a red cell is supposed to live for 120 days, can you survive the loss?

He answered that the body can regenerate half of its red cells in two days if it has to. But if it does, there will be elevated levels of two enzymes in the blood: alkaline phosphatase (alk phos) and lactic dehydrogenase (LDH). Alk phos and LDH are measured by blood profile enzyme tests.

Finally things began to fit together. Dr. Bowerman's comments on the enzymes fit with my oxygen-deficient anemia theory. Pulling all the bits of information together, this is what I had: If mercury attaches to hemoglobin so that it transports less oxygen; and if low oxygen content produces a compensatory increase in the number of red cells; and if the body rapidly replaces the red cells that have been contaminated with mercury, starting this whole chain of events; then blood tests should show elevated levels of these enzymes. I looked at patient chemistries before and after amalgam removal and saw this exact pattern emerge.

In acutely fatigued patients whose bone marrow is still working well at its job of producing red blood cells, I find elevated hemoglobin and hematocrit levels. Alk phos and LDH enzymes in the blood are elevated to the high normal range. Energy is low. After amalgam removal, the hemoglobin, hematocrit, and both enzymes decrease while the energy level increases.

Now I am quick to tell these "chronic fatigue" patients with high hemoglobin levels that it is *not* all in their heads. Well, maybe it is—but in the *lower* third of the head, not the upper third.

Long-term chronic fatigue is characterized by lower levels of hemoglobin and hematocrit, although these can still fall within the low normal range. This is because heavy metals such as mercury interfere with the production of the building blocks of the hemoglobin molecule itself. Mercury also interferes with the production of a substance called coenzyme A, which is necessary for the formation not only of hemoglobin, but of cholesterol as well. Now I have another link to observe.

Imagine this problem in combination with the fact that

mercury is cutting the efficiency of the hemoglobin that *is* there, and it is easy to see why the patient feels fatigued. Hemoglobin and hematocrit levels usually drop immediately after amalgam removal as the body rids itself of the faulty, inefficient hemoglobin, then they move upward after a few weeks. Energy is restored over a period of a few weeks, as compared to a few days in the patient with short-term fatigue.

### Urinary Mercury Excretion

When I started reading American articles on urinary excretion of mercury, the one consistent thing I found was inconsistency. Most of the medical and dental articles I read suggested that high levels of urinary mercury indicated toxicity, and conversely, that low levels indicated health. However . . . almost every article contained a "however" clause, such as: "However, we have seen people with high urinary mercury levels who were apparently in good health, and low levels in people who were sick."

None of these statements gave me confidence in their conclusions.

Urine levels of mercury have been interesting to study. Twenty years ago the articles on urinary excretion of mercury expressed puzzlement over the fact that some obviously mercury-toxic patients had high levels, while just as many had low levels. The general conclusion was that urinary mercury was meaningless.

After watching many urine reports and evaluating them along with the same patients' blood analyses and symptoms, a new idea was born. I noticed that those patients with low excretory levels of mercury were slower to respond to treatment than were those with higher levels. Then I noticed that a few patients had urine values that would suddenly skyrocket several thousand percent. These people generally showed faster recoveries than those whose urine levels moved very little.

To condense a long story of correlations, I came to the conclusion that people with low urine levels of mercury have *retention toxicity*. Should a person be exposed to, say, four units of mercury daily, and excrete four units daily, very little damage would be identified. Should that person suddenly experience some biological change such that his or her excretion dropped to two units excreted for every four units of exposure, mercury would start to accumulate, and when his or her biological threshold was reached, symptoms related to retention toxicity could develop. This provided me with a logical biological answer, but not the simple one I had hoped for.

What I found in the literature regarding toxic levels of mercury sounded more like an auction than scientific proof of levels of toxicity. Dentistry (which had the most to lose from the establishment of a low figure) came onto the scene with its guesses. Dr. Wilmer Eames bid 150 micrograms of mercury per liter of urine, but was overshadowed by P.L. Fan, D.D.S., of the ADA, who "established" (with no research or publications) 500 micrograms as the safe upper limit. Again I took my dilemma to Dr. David Bowerman. He told me to call the Centers for Disease Control (CDC) in Atlanta, Georgia. When an epidemic strikes, the CDC is our primary defense. When Legionnaires' disease hit, for instance, the CDC was called first. It was the logical call to make.

I contacted a toxicologist at the CDC and asked who had the ultimate responsibility for setting the standards of safety and toxicity in the United States. He said that the CDC did. I asked him at what level mercury in urine was considered reflective of toxicity. He answered that it was 30 micrograms per liter.

I asked if dentistry was within CDC jurisdiction. I was told that dentistry is a self-policing profession with high ethical standards, and as such was not directly responsible to CDC, or anyone else for that matter. He said that dentistry ultimately is responsible for itself.

I then told him of the floating 150- to 500-microgram safety limit that was being advertised by dentistry. He was rather attentive. I asked him for a quotable comment about the dental proclamations. He readily replied, "It looks to me like an accommodation for sloppy procedures."

I decided to start testing urine samples for mercury to see what effect, if any, amalgam removal procedures would have. Using scientific personal disinterest as a guide, I selected for testing the next patient to come in for mercury detoxification. Her urinary excretion was 12 micrograms per liter. I retested her, using another sample, to see how variable she might be. The next test showed 10 micrograms. Then, after amalgam removal, her excretion shot up to 136 micrograms. Also notable were her other test results. Her white blood cell count dropped from a three-year average of 17,500 to 10,500. Her body temperature went from high 96s and low 97s to 98.6°F. All of that took place in one day after amalgam removal.

After several years' experience of monitoring urine mercury, today I believe that 4 to 8 micrograms per liter in the urine reflects the body ridding itself of routine daily exposures from air, food, and water. Levels below that suggest either no mercury exposure (rare on this planet), or a reduced ability to excrete mercury.

Patients with the most severe symptoms seem to fall into the category of lower than 4 micrograms of excretion. I rarely get these patients to make quantum leaps like the first patient did. But I do note that at these low levels a patient will start making perceptible progress when the excretion goes up 100 percent. That is, a person with 1 microgram would have to increase to 2 micrograms; a person with 2 micrograms would have to progress to 4 micrograms. After 4 micrograms, the percentage is not as important, but it certainly is an indicator at the very low levels.

After watching patient progress relative to urine mercury, I decided that my term *retention toxicity* really did describe the patient who is mercury toxic because of a lack of ability to excrete. When the original blueprint of man was drawn, there was mercury on the planet. People probably had the ability to excrete it then, and some do today. My observations suggest that the mercury-toxic patient loses some ability to excrete mercury when amalgam is placed in his or her mouth. That assumption is based on observing so many patients who had very little in the way of health problems until amalgam was placed. Upon removal of the amalgam, they excreted more mercury, and their symptoms improved. In a few of these patients, some improvements were noted after half of their amalgams were removed. Most, however, have to have the last fleck removed before they start improving.

After amalgam removal, the problem of retention toxicity can be confronted—that is, if the fillings are removed sequentially; if compatible materials are used; if nutritional guidelines are followed, and more. If not, it is really tough to correct retention toxicity.


## Electrical Current

One of the most important techniques used in correcting the problems of mercury toxicity may not even be fully understood for quite some time. It remains highly significant nonetheless. After some ten months of using an electrical meter called an ammeter to chart positive and negative electrical currents on fillings, I found by accident that these different currents had meaning. At that time, only 10 to 15 percent of my patients were responding well to amalgam removal. But when I observed those who had their high negative-current fillings removed first, I found that low response shot up to over 50 percent.

Fred Lerner, B.S., M.S., D.C., Ph.D., who has a degree in bioelectricity, recently told me he had a plausible idea regarding the reactions I have seen. He told me that a negative-current filling would be pushing electrons into the body, and that the positive-current fillings would be acting as a sump, or area where the electrons exited the body. Removing a positive filling is like shutting off a water faucet quickly. All the pipes in the house rattle (just as all the nerves would rattle) if the exit sump is shut off suddenly. It made sense to him. All I know is that chemistries and symptoms make better improvements when the negative-current fillings are removed first.

I also know that electrical current is a measurement of the speed of a chemical reaction. From this I could assume that the higher the current, the more mercury vapor is being released from the filling.

Electrical current, or oral galvanism as it was called years ago, is not new to discussions in medicine and dentistry. As discussed in Chapter 2, publications from J.J.R. Patrick back in 1880 mentioned oral galvanism. After reading Dr. Pinto's 1976 publication, I noted almost unanimous agreement in writings from 1940 by E.S. Lain, W. Schriever, and G.S. Caughron that:

1. The human saliva constitutes a good electrolyte (a substance capable of conducting electricity).
2. In every oral cavity containing dissimilar metals all the elements of galvanic cells (areas that produce electricity) are present.
3. Certain symptoms and pathologic lesions in the

mouth diagnosed as electrogalvanic lesions disappear after complete and direct replacement of amalgams with certain metals.

Lain and Caughron together wrote over thirty articles on the medical dangers of electrical current in the mouth due to fillings. In 1941, I.C. Schoonover and W. Sounder investigated the rate of corrosion of dental amalgam under various conditions and stated in an August 1941 article in the *Journal of the American Dental Association*:

> One has only to examine the surface and base of any dental fillings to observe corrosion, which is probably the result of galvanic action. Such amalgams need not be in contact with other metal or in mouths containing additional metal fillings.
>
> Galvanic action on a single metal filling may also result from exposure of different areas of the filling to solutions that are not chemically the same. Such a condition produces a simple concentration cell, which in dental practice would be found where an amalgam restoration fails to seal the cavity. The base of such an amalgam would be exposed to a solution of a different concentration, for example of oxygen, from that in contact with the surface.

Well, a lot has happened for me since those days of stumbling around with a meter, pad, and pencil. Clinical observation soon taught me that most people with severe cases of MS, epilepsy, or emotional disease had lots of negative-current fillings. They usually had six or more. About 15 percent had fewer than six negative fillings and about 5 percent had no negatives, so electrical current is not diagnostic, but the trend shows through.

This puzzling finding on electrical current is the difference between success and failure in some cases. If the negative fillings are removed first, the patient's chances of improving are good. If the positively charged fillings are removed first, leaving the negative behind, chances for success drop substantially. Now, the dentist does not have to jump around all over the mouth chasing current. As mentioned previously, I have noticed that if all of the fillings are removed from the quadrant (one-quarter of the mouth) with the highest negative readings first, the patient will have a reasonable chance of getting well. After all the quadrants with negative fillings are completed, then those with high positive current are removed. Following this sequence—called sequential amalgam removal—has proven to be a very effective way of removing fillings. I still have a number of patients who heard about mercury toxicity, ran out and had their fillings removed at random, and have yet to show any improvement. This is a very technical, sensitive procedure. Don't hurt yourself through haste.

Looking back at the 1970s now, I know why my patients responded only 10 percent of the time. At the time, I always removed fillings by starting in the upper left quadrant, just because that's where I had *always* started. There was no science to it, just a habit. Possibly, by sheer coincidence, about one time in ten I treated a patient whose highest negative current was in the upper left quadrant.

Electrical current is generated on the surface of single fillings, between two fillings that touch, and between the filling and the dentinal fluid beneath the filling. That makes for complexity.

What does it mean if you touch a tooth with the probe of an ammeter and the meter doesn't show a reading, negative or positive? This means that the filling is either pure gold (gold foils usually do not register current); that it is a low-metallic-volume composite (which usually doesn't have a current unless Dycal is used as a base under the filling); or that it is an amalgam that is highly corroded.

When a filling has undergone heavy corrosion, there is a layer of corroded material on the outer surface. Often a probe cannot get through this layer even when the filling is scratched. If this is the case, I recommend that a dental bur be used to spot polish the filling so that the probe can get past the corrosion layer. In about 80 percent of the cases, I find these highly corroded fillings to be negative. Is it possible that negative current, in addition to being related to higher production of methyl mercury (see page 31), is also related to higher corrosion rates? What type of relationship really exists here?

There are a few things that appear to be extremely important about dental materials and electrical current. The first is that gold and amalgam should not be in the mouth at the same time. If they are, the amount of electrical current increases tremendously, and can lead to severe problems in susceptible people. If you are having your amalgams replaced with gold, all amalgam should be removed first, and then the gold crowns should be placed. (You can have plastic temporary crowns placed until all the amalgam has been removed.) Under no circumstances would I now put gold in a mouth that contains amalgam.

What is considered high current in the mouth? Reinhold Voll, M.D., of Germany, recommends against the presence of more than 4 microamps of current. He suggests that greater amounts of current affect the acupuncture meridians in the body adversely and contribute to disease processes. You can think of these meridians as violin strings running from the top of the body through the teeth and to the bottom of the feet. I myself am concerned about negative current at *any* level. I feel that the dramatic improvements I have seen in some of my patients are due to the removal of their electrical current field, in addition to getting rid of the mercury.

Gold crowns can have very high electrical currents, but they are seldom negative. If the gold alloy (crowns are not made of pure gold because it is too soft) contains copper, the current can be quite high. I usually do not recommend that these be removed unless you still have symptoms that have not cleared up after all amalgam has been out of the mouth for a few weeks.

The last thing I would like to note about electrical current in regard to treatment is the case of the suicidal patient. If there is a lot of negative current, it may be wise to replace only half of the amalgam in the first quadrant during the first appointment. The suicidal patient is extremely sensitive to changes in electrical current. I strongly recommend that such a patient be given protamine zinc insulin (PZI) in the area of the amalgam removal at each appointment, and that this patient have someone with him or her at all times for the first twenty-four hours after the procedure. PZI has a calming effect on a person's emotions. The primary action of PZI is to increase circulation and stimulate formation of new blood vessels around the area of injection. Its precise mechanisms are not totally understood, but the positive effects have become obvious through clinical observation.

As you can see, electrical current is a very important aspect of treatment for mercury toxicity. I hope to understand more about the hows and whys of electrical current as time goes by. But in the meantime, I again want to caution you against having your fillings removed in random order. Sequential amalgam removal is a must for the patient with multiple or severe symptoms. (See Chapter 7.)

## Questionnaire

Questionnaires are not exactly diagnostic tools in themselves, but they can surely point the doctor in the right direction to find diagnostic data. I use an extensive questionnaire that examines problems in lifestyle and in carbohydrate, protein, and fat intake; shows symptoms and signs that are frequently associated with specific chemical imbalances; and occasionally uncovers surprises.

Questionnaires are interesting tests. They give information on a patient's current status, but more than that, they can educate an observer. I'm not sure where this education is headed, but I am noticing trends in symptoms. I have noted, for instance, that people with numbness and tingling in their fingers and toes have low manganese levels. Given long enough, they can end up with MS-like symptoms. If they have numbness and MS, they eventually can have heart irregularities and emotional problems. From there they can proceed to fatigue and a series of hormonal disturbances that may be related to sulfur-bond interference. If this information could be combined with patient chemistries, I might find ways to push my success rate even higher.

The analyses discussed in this chapter—blood profile, hair, CBC, urine mercury, electrical current, and the questionnaire—give sufficient data to allow a trained clinician to diagnose and plan treatment for the average mercury-toxic patient. A lot can be done even for severe cases of epilepsy, arthritis, allergies, and the other diseases mentioned throughout this book. But there is always more. Perfection is always a step away. There are unending numbers of frontiers to explore.

## OTHER FACTORS IN DIAGNOSIS

There are many other tests that are not universally significant, but that allow a better understanding of the disease process in selected individuals. In this section I will discuss some of those interesting tidbits that become major players in treating some people.

## Seven–Fourteen–Twenty-One–Day Immune Cycle

The seven–fourteen–twenty-one–day immune cycle has proven to be a major factor in almost all cases. The day that the immune system receives a challenge, like the placement of a silver-mercury amalgam filling, becomes day one of a predictable cycle of events. I have observed that seven days from that day, if another immune challenge (like the placement of another filling) occurs, the patient will feel like he is coming down with the flu for a couple of hours. Then he will feel okay again and forget about the reaction. If another seven days go by—the fourteenth day since the original challenge—and an immune challenge occurs, the patient may come down with "whatever is going around" for a day or two. Should a challenge occur on the twenty-first day from the original placement of a filling, the person's genetic weak link may break, and a really serious autoimmune disease can appear. I first observed this in a person who had a really bad case of the flu. He had an amalgam placed twenty-one days later, and he immediately began to experience symptoms that eventually led to MS.

Over the past ten years, I have seen countless cases of this cycle appearing to be related to disease onset. Now I am hearing similar stories related to chemotherapy. The scenario goes like this: Chemotherapy is administered. The patient experiences nausea, vomiting, hair loss, and an assorted flurry of side effects. Twenty-one days later, the patient again experiences nausea, vomiting, hair loss, and an assorted flurry of side effects. The sequence of events is duplicated except for one thing: The second time there was no chemotherapy, just the side effects.

What happens? White blood cells, like all cells in your body, live a cyclical existence. Seven, fourteen, and twenty-one days after a challenge, legions of your little defense soldiers are dying off while new, inexperienced recruits are being brought in. During the changing of the guard, there is a time of reduced defense. Herein lies your susceptibility.

A man called recently to tell me that a cancer therapy was working on his wife. It had been so successful that he had been asked to write a book on the success story. After being told she was totally cured—a grapefruit-sized tumor had completely dissolved—she was given a booster (twenty-one days from the last treatment), and suddenly, without any apparent reason, she died.

The moral of the story is to avoid those low-defense days in making appointments with your dentist. In my office, I have a patient come in for two weeks. Dental appointments may be scheduled on Monday, Wednesday, and Friday the first week, then finish on either Tuesday or Thursday of the next week. I tell patients to take it easy on the twenty-first day from each of the initial dental appointments. These are not the days to plan a fifty-mile hike or any sort of out-of-the-ordinary physically or emotionally stressful event. Many people will feel the second twenty-one-day cycle symptoms—which are usually mild, but similar to the original symptoms that drove you to consider amalgam removal in the first place—at forty-two days, and seriously ill patients will note a drop in energy even at sixty-three days.

## Psychological Testing

As I mentioned in Chapter 2, in 1976 a psychologist from the University of Colorado said, in essence, that people process thought differently with amalgams than they do after amalgam removal. He said that people cope better without their amalgams. He had devised a test to measure the psychological states of people before and after amalgam removal. I ran out of money to continue the study, but now have enough suggestions to keep a graduate student busy for years trying to put together the brain connections that we have observed.

Some people have spoken to psychiatrists for years, with little visible progress. After amalgam removal, they are far more capable of addressing and processing their problems to completion.

Many patients have been emotionally or physically abused as children. They have no conscious memory of these events at all—until the first quadrant of high-negative fillings comes out. Sometimes while still in the dental chair they view a full-color replay of those forgotten events. Wow, what reactions they can have. The poor dentist is usually unaware of what is going on. My patients are forewarned of these possibilities, and I have three people on staff trained to help these patients to a soft, safe landing. They are not psychologically "cured" at that moment, but direction and explanation are provided, so that they can get help back home to complete the process so they can live a more normal existence.

Psychological changes have been the most interesting segment of healing that I have witnessed. You never know how people are going to handle these events. I still recoil in horror at some of the stories patients tell me, but the vast majority of them are tremendously relieved to find out what has caused their problems.

Dr. Jaro Pleva, relating his experiences in 1983, when physicians were unable to help him with his complaints and health problems, said in a September 1983 article in the *Journal of Orthomolecular Psychiatry*:

The diagnosis that all this was because of stress or strained relations in the family I could not take seriously. From my previous life I was used to more stress, both psychic and physical, than during this period.

About five months after the last amalgam filling had been removed some relatively strong symptoms returned for a period of one to two weeks. After this period I had a feeling of even better well-being than before.

The improvements in my health could not be related to any factor in my surroundings. Finally I want to stress the amazing improvement in well-being, only three months after the final dental treatment. In spite of still improving, I have regained a feeling of peace and calmness, of being able to appreciate smells, details, and graduations in my surroundings, something I must go back 10–15 years to find.

In his list of symptoms in his article, he described his emotional and psychological problems as being those of severe amnesia, constant strain, anxiety, irritability, difficulty in, and even inability to control, behavior, indecision, loss of interest in life, tiredness, and aging. Within weeks of amalgam removal, his emotional balance was back to normal and he was happy again.

### Body Temperature

Mercury-toxic patients frequently have a low body temperature, because chances are there is mercury blocking the thyroid hormone. The thyroid hormone has four activation sites (little binding sites, as they are called in the profession) onto which iodine can attach. When mercury occupies one of these positions, iodine cannot hook up with them. If the thyroid hormone has iodine in these positions, it is an active hormone. If anything other than iodine is there, the thyroid hormone does not behave properly. Mercury gets into these activation positions and never lets go. As a result, even though a "thyroid function test" indicates available thyroid hormone, the mercury on the iodine positions prevents the thyroid from reacting as it should.

Usually within twenty-four hours of final amalgam removal, body temperature has moved toward 98.6°F. It may not make it all the way in one day, but even 96s and 97s can get into the 98° category. There is bound to be a hormonal problem involved, but which one and how much? Only testing will tell for sure. But the real question is, Does dentistry have the right to place something in your mouth that lowers your body temperature one or two degrees?

### Fundus Photography of the Retina

The eyes have it—mercury. Doty Murphy, M.D., called several years ago to ask if I had an ophthalmoscope, an instrument used to look at the retina in the back of the eyeball. I didn't have one, but the fellow next door did. When I looked through it, all I could positively identify was my eyelash.

Dr. Murphy described black streaks that occur in the retina. The medical profession considers these to be areas where the elongated near-sighted eye has put tension on the retina and stretched it so that the epithelium (the layer of tissue below the retina) shows through. Dr. Murphy, however, had noted that these occurred in people who had amalgam in their mouths, and were absent in people without amalgam. Another strange thing is that when amalgams are removed, the black areas begin to disappear. I now have some progress photographs to demonstrate this.

Dentists see black spots, too. In the mouth they are called "amalgam tattoos." They supposedly occur when the dentist (the sloppy one across the street, not yours) slips with the drill and cuts up the gums slightly. Then when he places the amalgam, he inadvertently presses some of it into the cut tissue, and doesn't wash it out. What you see is the amalgam "tattooed" into the tissues.

That explanation satisfied me until I found amalgam tattoos in the roof of the mouth, down the bony ridge an inch away from a lower tooth, and finally—the one that did it—on the uvula. The uvula is that little finger-like projection that hangs down at the very back of your soft palate. Convince me that a dentist hit that with a drill and then smeared amalgam into it! There aren't enough sloppy dentists to account for the number of amalgam tattoos I see.

Do you suppose those dark areas in the retina are amalgam tattoos? Do they affect vision? Some people think they do. Ask around. Do you have an astigmatism? When did you start wearing glasses for myopia (nearsightedness)? When did you get your first amalgams? Were the two developments within six months of each other? Some optometrists feel that myopia and cataracts are related to mercury in fish and amalgam. Research is being done in these areas as well.

Yes, all of these are new frontiers. They can all potentially tell us a lot about the ways in which mercury and other heavy metals can affect us biologically. I would encourage our scientists and university researchers to begin earnest work in as many of these areas as possible.

Poking a balloon with a pin will break the balloon, but pulling the pin out will not restore it. Such is the case with mercury toxicity. A filling placed during a thirty-minute dental appointment can push you over the threshold, but removing that filling does not put you together again. Since mercury has its choice—directed by your genetic susceptibility—as to where to disturb your metabolism, where the damage will occur is unpredictable. How much damage it will do—again genetically controlled—is impossible to predict, and how fast you can recover is in the same category.

There are things you can do to help your body, however. You can find a trained dentist to replace your fillings sequentially. You can have them replaced with "compatible" dental materials. You can avoid the seven–fourteen–twenty-one–day immune cycle trap. Further, you can prepare your body for all this with proper diet and supplementation.

Notice the word "you." It appears frequently. Yes, *you* will have to become responsible for seeing that these things are done, because most dentists do not have the time to do them for you unless you insist.

# 7

# Recovering From Mercury Toxicity

*I* hope you now have a clear understanding of the severity of mercury toxicity and the need for a properly planned treatment regimen. I have mentioned sequential amalgam removal, and in this chapter I will tell you exactly what it is, how it's done, and where you can get it.

## GETTING STARTED

The first step toward recovery from mercury toxicity is to have your amalgams removed. As I have mentioned, however, you shouldn't just run out to the nearest dentist and ask him to take out your fillings. Instead, try to follow the sequence of procedures below as closely as possible.

First, if you're uncertain that mercury is a problem, have the urine porphyrin test run. Remember, mercury is the only heavy metal that causes a blockage in the conversion of body-formed chemicals called porphyrins into hemoglobin and the energy storage unit called ATP. Blocking this process robs your body of energy needed for repair and normal activity. This blockage also causes the porphyrins to accumulate in the blood until they spill over into the urine. If your urine shows high levels, it is pretty obvious that mercury is causing you a problem. To find a dentist who will perform this test, call the Huggins Diagnostic Center.

Next, have an electrical reading of your amalgams done. If this is not available in your area, contact my office for a referral. An electrical current reading gives a general idea of the speed of electrochemical reactions occurring on the surface of the fillings. It also reflects the conditions that encourage conversion of ordinarily toxic mercury into the horribly toxic methyl mercury. The higher the amperage reading in the negative electrical mode, the more conducive the environment is to the conversion of mercury into methyl mercury.

Positive charges on fillings do not indicate safety; they just indicate that poisons are being released at a slower rate. They still require removal where healing is desired.

Electrical charge readings change over a period of hours or days because these areas on the fillings are "dynamic," or highly reactive electrically. Just chewing gum or having vinegar (acidic) and oil dressing on a salad can clear off a microlayer of corrosion and change the fillings' electrical activity. Once the process of amalgam removal is begun, removing a few fillings will alter the components of the battery, resulting in changing current. For most people, these daily fluctuations are not great enough to be significant until after a week or so, but this is not true for people with leukemia or ALS. These folks respond when the fillings are removed in absolute sequence—that is in descending order, from high negatives to low positives, such as in -12, -9, -2, +20, +10, +3. This means the dentist may be jumping from an upper tooth to a lower tooth, from right to left, in a time-consuming pattern, but the results have been decisive. Neither of these diseases falls into the totally reversible category, but when the absolute sequence is used, I frequently see improvements. When fillings are not removed this way—even though all other procedures are followed—there is no interruption in the downward progression of the disease.

Third, have basic testing completed—CBC, blood chemistry profile, hair analysis, and urine mercury—if you have any symptoms or problems at all and are planning to proceed with treatment. If you have no health problems, but are removing amalgams only for preventative reasons, you may be able to skip the testing, but be sure that you have the electrical readings done for sequential removal, and be sure to have your fillings replaced with compatible dental materials.

If you do have blood testing done, remember that it is the interpretation that counts, not the numerical value. Sometimes a high white blood cell count means a bad infection is getting the best of you, which is bad (you need antibiotics), but that same numerical figure can indicate that your immune system is already winning the battle and antibiotics would hinder your progress.

How can you tell if you make progress? Only through the use of "before" and "after" chemistries can you know where you have been and where you are headed. Follow-up chemistries can inform you and your doctor of under-correction, proper treatment, or overcorrection. They can be valuable.

Fourth, start dietary supplementation as determined by test results at least one or two weeks before amalgam removal. According to what I see in follow-up urine mercury excretion, as well as symptom and chemistry response, supplementation seems to condition the body to excrete unwanted mercury and to begin tissue repair. Excretion of both methyl mercury and inorganic mercury tends to increase if supplementation is started several days prior to amalgam removal.

Even if blood chemistry analysis is not used as a guide to plan treatment for an individual patient, I have found a couple of nutritional supplements that can benefit the patient without creating imbalances. These are TransMix (a multimineral form that appears to improve the efficiency of cell membranes), Eater's Digest (a digestive enzyme), and vitamin C. I *do* use other supplementation, but specific supplements and their dosages are based on the excesses and deficiencies shown in individual blood chemistries. They are not used unless they are needed. TransMix, Eater's Digest, and vitamin C are good for pre-treatment as well as for maintenance afterwards. One note of caution, however. Do not take vitamin C the morning of a dental appointment. C erases much of the effect of the anesthetic and you may experience *pain*. (Taking it afterwards is fine.) Should you forget this tidbit, consider the result a learning experience.

Finally, before having your amalgams removed, you *must* have a serum compatibility test run so that your replacement fillings will not cause you more damage than your amalgam fillings. This is available through your dentist, or can be ordered directly through Huggins Diagnostic Center. There are actually plastic fillings (called composites) and insulative bases that go under them that can set off different health problems from what amalgam gave you. These may not be as life-threatening as mercury from the toxic standpoint, but consider this: Many of the composites contain aluminum. Aluminum is suspected in mental disorders. The most common mental upset I see is suicidal thoughts. These folks do not often actually commit suicide, but the thoughts hound them most of their waking hours. Is this a worthwhile trade-off?

Other important considerations are:

- Do not have crowns permanently cemented for at least one month after amalgam removal if your symptoms are severe.
- Do not use bases like Dycal.
- Avoid other mercury exposures (see Chapter 8).
- Avoid having all appointments on the same day of the week, in order to avoid interfering with the seven–fourteen–twenty-one–day immune cycle.
- If suicidal thoughts are among your symptoms, be sure PZI (protamine zinc insulin) is used with each quadrant of amalgam that is removed, and have someone stay with you for the first twenty-four hours after treatment. The more negative-current fillings you have, the more important this is.

If you are unable to find someone who can plan your treatment, and are unable to come to my office, I can still help you with a computer program designed specifically for this purpose. I can refer you to dentists in your area who are willing to help. You may contact my office for further information. There should be no reason for anyone suffering from mercury toxicity to be unable to find help.


## THE BUBBLE-OPERATORY

In 1973, I quit placing amalgam fillings. Patient protection was a big concern, but I didn't want the daily personal exposure either. My mercury-toxic mind and I then continued cutting old silver-mercury amalgams out of people's mouths for eleven more years, not once thinking that I was taking a shower bath in mercury mist for several hours every day.

Duane Cutright, D.D.S., Ph.D., in his article, "Systemic

Mercury Levels Caused by Inhaling Mist During High-speed Amalgam Grinding," describes increases in mercury levels in a dentist's brain, heart, liver, and kidneys after ten-minute exposures to cutting amalgam. This started me thinking about a safe dental operatory. After a six-year gestation period, the first prototype of a new dental operatory—the bubble-operatory—that is safe for the patient, doctor, and assistant was born.

Since fillings generate electrical current, and all electricity has some effect on the body, I decided to incorporate this knowledge into the bubble-op concept. I started with a Faraday cage. This is a fine wire mesh that encases the walls and ceilings and is attached to grounding rods that reach several meters into the soil. Next I added an electronic mercury-particle and vapor removing device, and two high-powered air filters with a combination of filtering materials that I researched and designed. The corners and floor-to-ceiling angles were rounded for better control of air flow; hence the name bubble-op was coined to describe the bubble-shaped operatory. Dialysis tubing (assumed to be free of contaminants and heavy metals because of the delicate nature of dialysis) replaced normal plastic tubing; a deionizing water processor was used for water delivery; and materials that emitted no gases into the air were used for the floor, cabinets, and walls.

Paints were tested with a mercury vapor detector to make sure I did not have an unknown source of mercury. Three of the five "mercury-free" paints I tested emitted high levels of mercury vapor. Air mercury vapor tests and particulate counts showed that I had good control over the air. The amount of mercury vapor in the air during active procedures dropped from 880 micrograms per cubic meter without the system functioning to zero when it was fully functional.

Now that I am into the second- and third-generation bubble-op, I am observing healing that is beyond what I saw in conventional dental offices. Has it been worth the fuss and bustle of unconventional construction? You bet it has.

## NUTRITIONAL NECESSITIES

Taking out fillings is a necessary first step if one wants to recover from the ravages of mercury toxicity, but it is far from the only step. Nutrition is actually the most important component in restoring your body.

Improper nutrition destroys more recoveries than anything else, except for overdoing things once you start feeling better. It seems that there are more ways to injure the human body than to fix it. Changing our nutritional habits is fine for a few weeks, but then, when we are feeling better, that feeling of immortality comes over us again, and we return to our old habits. I spend a lot of time being outrageous in any way I can to get my patients' attention so they really learn about nutrition. After all, your old dietary habits probably set you up to get sick in the first place, and a return to eating the old way is going to reward you with the same old problems again.

I personally understand eating habits. I also know the arguments. I keep telling my father that he is going to have to get off those Post Toasties. He eats them daily. Anything you eat daily you are apt to become sensitized to, and he is taking a chance. After all, he started eating them daily when he was four years old. He is now eighty-six and doing fine, but one of these days an allergy due to frequent exposure is going to get him.

We all have relatives or friends who defy dietary good sense and get away with it. There are lots of arguments about nutrition. How do you know what to do? I have found that balancing body chemistry by letting your blood test report direct me to your ancestral diet consistently offers the best results.

It was noted by Dr. Weston Price and Melvin Page, D.D.S., decades ago that balancing chemistry through proper nutrition was the primary significant step in recovery from any disease. Both gentlemen studied thousands of patients from a nutritional point of view. Dr. Price traveled the world several times during the 1920s and 1930s to study primitive diets and the effects of "foods of commerce."

How do I find your ancestral diet? I watch your chemistry. How much protein do you need? Enough to keep your serum "total protein" level between 6.8 and 7.2 grams per 100 milliliters of blood serum. What about carbohydrates and fats? It's the same thing. There are levels of these chemistries that reappear in most folks when their biochemistry is reflective of their ancestral diet.

### Eight Blood Tests

All blood tests are important, but there are eight that tell more of your basic story than any others. Let's spend some time discussing these primary chemistries, which include combinations of phosphorous, glucose, cholesterol, triglycerides, total protein, globulin, lactic dehydrogenase (LDH), and alkaline phosphatase (alk phos).

*Phosphorous.* The relative balance of the endocrine system is reflected by the serum phosphorous level. When it is low, I know there is a hormonal disturbance somewhere, but I don't know exactly where it is. In the days when I was doing only body chemistry (nutritional and biochemical counseling), I had to look at several different hormone levels if dietary corrections failed to help. Today, I see quite rapid improvement in hormonal disturbances once amalgam removal has been completed. This assumes that dietary factors are also being addressed simultaneously.

Dietary factors that lower the phosphorus level tend to raise the level of three other substances: glucose, cholesterol, and triglycerides. It becomes necessary, then, to avoid chemicals that cause this alteration. These are primarily sugar, alcohol, and caffeine. Any time these items are in the diet, there will be a drop in phosphorus and a simultaneous endocrine imbalance, as they interfere with the production of hormones by the endocrine glands. Sugar, alcohol, and caffeine push the glucose, cholesterol, and triglycerides up; then the endocrine function is slowed, and the phosphorus level is pushed down.

One of the things I watch to help identify the mercury-toxic patient is the relationship between glucose and cholesterol. I look first at the glucose level. If it is elevated, I then look to cholesterol. Where dietary infractions are elevating the glucose, the cholesterol will usually be elevated also. But if the cholesterol is lower than its ideal level while the glucose is elevated, then I suspect mercury interference with the body's ability to form cholesterol.

*Glucose.* A glucose test is a measurement of the blood sugar level. The body converts nearly all the food we eat into glucose, because it is a necessary fuel for life. But when the glucose remains continuously elevated, many tissues are constantly bathed in it, which is very unhealthy. For example, by the use of an instrument called a Peritron, I can determine the amount of glucose in the fluid that surrounds the tooth. Persons with high levels of glucose in the blood also show high glucose in the fluid surrounding each tooth. Those with high glucose in the fluid show greater amounts of periodontal disease than those with ideal levels. There is a direct relationship in that the higher the glucose, the more severe the gum disease.

Glucose in the body acts to provide adequate energy. If it is maintained at an even, moderate level, the energy level remains constant. The entire body depends upon a sufficient, but not overly abundant, supply of glucose. If something elevates the glucose sharply, the biological systems become overloaded. At this point, the pancreas detects the elevation and produces insulin to "burn up" the excess glucose, because the body has been designed to run at an even level known as homeostasis. When this equilibrium is disturbed, the entire body is affected. In my experience, elevations in glucose levels indicate the beginnings of degenerative diseases—those that gradually wear the body down. Examples are arthritis, diabetes, and high blood pressure. To help avoid these diseases, it is best to keep the glucose level under control.

Many things can elevate the glucose level. All drugs, whether prescription or over-the-counter, can elevate it. But I am primarily interested here in nutritional influences. Sugar, alcohol, caffeine, and fruit juices are the most influential factors in altering glucose levels. Sugar and fruit juices do most of their damage because they are what Dr. Weston Price termed *partitioned foods*. This means that they have been partially stripped of the vitamins, minerals, and enzymes that enable the body to metabolize them, or break them down. These elements are primarily in the pulp, which is thrown away. The sugar in juice is dumped headlong into the glucose metabolic pathway, and is very quickly transformed into glucose, thus elevating a person's glucose level and causing the body to have to compensate for it. Having foods and drinks with sugar in them is like repeatedly racing your car up to 150 miles per hour and then slamming on the brakes. The more you do this to your car, the sooner it will wear out. Insulin production is analogous to slamming on the brakes.

Alcohol, caffeine, and fruit juices all have the same

effect on blood glucose. I caution all diabetics to avoid not only sugar, but caffeine as well. One cup of coffee can elevate the glucose level enough to require three units of insulin to counteract it. Yet most diabetics consume more than one cup of a caffeine-containing beverage per day, thus increasing their insulin requirements.

There are other factors that must be in balance to maintain an ideal glucose level. Certain minerals are necessary to activate the enzyme systems involved in glucose metabolism. One of these is chromium, which works to increase the permeability of the cell membrane, and to enable the glucose to get into the cell instead of remaining in the bloodstream or in the fluids around the cell. A deficiency of chromium can be caused by consuming too much refined carbohydrate, such as sugar, alcohol, and white flour.

Zinc is a mineral that is a part of the insulin molecule itself. When zinc is deficient, production of insulin may not be adequate to control glucose, especially if you eat a high-carbohydrate diet. In addition to deactivating the insulin molecule, mercury also plays a part in causing zinc deficiency.

Manganese also helps to control the glucose level, as does magnesium. The excretion of both of these minerals is hastened by the diuretic effect of alcohol and caffeine, offering yet another reason why alcohol and caffeine cause an elevated glucose level.

Finally, vitamin C is necessary in the control of glucose. Anything that destroys vitamin C can potentially increase glucose, including cigarettes, stress, drugs, and dietary factors.

What can you do to be certain that you are not interfering with the action of the treatment for mercury toxicity to lower blood glucose? Avoid sugar, alcohol, and caffeine. Fruit juice and refined carbohydrates should be limited to amounts that

do not interfere with your phosphorus, glucose, cholesterol, and triglycerides. To make up for these items, eat
more protein, like turkey and beef. Avoid partitioned and
overcooked foods, and avoid tobacco products.

*Cholesterol.* High levels of cholesterol are caused primarily by the consumption of sugar, alcohol, and caffeine.
Recent weight loss, stress, insufficient thyroid function,
tobacco, drugs (especially antihistamines), and low levels
of certain minerals (chromium, magnesium, calcium, and
manganese) are other causes. Did you notice that not once
in this list did I mention any food that contains cholesterol,
such as eggs and butter? This is because these things will
not raise your cholesterol level if you keep sugar, alcohol,
and caffeine out of your diet. Sugar raises cholesterol
perhaps more than anything else; therefore, control of
cholesterol is impossible when sugar is in the diet. Many
patients who were once on medication to lower their
cholesterol have been able to eliminate completely their
need for drugs by controlling their diets.

Normally, when sugar, alcohol, or caffeine is in the diet,
glucose and cholesterol are both elevated. In the mercury-
toxic patient, I may find elevated glucose with deficient
cholesterol. Many body functions are affected when this is
the case. If we do not get cholesterol through dietary intake,
the body will produce its own because of the importance of
this raw material. In fact, 80 percent of all cholesterol in the
blood serum is produced by the body from foods that do not
contain cholesterol. What functions could be so important?
One area of interest to nearly everyone who would like to
lose weight is that ingested fats enable nutrients to be absorbed. Since *true* hunger is the body's search for nutrients,
fats play an important role in preventing this hunger, because all nutrients are absorbed best in conjunction with fat.
These nutrients—amino acids, fatty acids, vitamins, and

minerals—are necessary to rebuild body tissues. A lack of fat reduces the body's absorption of everything except calories, so in many cases a lack of adequate fat in the diet is actually related to the buildup of fatty deposits. The addition of fat to the diet makes it possible for the body to pick up nutrients efficiently, so it doesn't have to keep asking for more of them by becoming hungry. This is contrary to what many people think, but the truth of it has been demonstrated by the thousands of people who have gone on this type of diet.

The amount of fat, as well as of carbohydrates and proteins, that an individual needs is determined by watching blood chemistry. There is no one standard amount for all people. Rather, your genetic inheritance determines how much of each you need to keep these three areas of blood chemistry in balance. So weight control is dependent upon the proper fats in the diet, assuming, of course, that sugar, alcohol, and caffeine are out of the diet.

Cholesterol is found in the myelinated nerve sheath, which is the protective layer that insulates the nerves against erratic electric charges. Lack of this nerve sheath is one of the problems with the MS patient.

Cholesterol is necessary for proper brain function. More than 10 percent of the dry weight of the brain is composed of cholesterol.

Cholesterol is part of the insulation layer around the heart, so proper dietary fats help to protect against heart disease and traumatic injuries.

Cholesterol is necessary for the manufacture and transport of the sex hormones testosterone and estrogen, so it is important that, during puberty, youngsters have sufficient amounts of healthy fats (butter rather than margarine, for example) in order to have the raw materials required for proper sexual maturation.

Cholesterol is necessary as a raw material needed in the production of energy in the red blood cells.

One-fourth of all the enzyme systems are dependent upon fats, and upon absorption of nutrients through the intestines via fat solubility. Therefore, all of the enzymes involved in the cell membrane transport system are cholesterol-dependent. This is important because if you do not have proper cell membrane transport (the ability to get nutrients into, and manufactured products out of, the cells), then you are not getting the benefit of the minerals you are consuming, whether by supplement or in your food.

Cholesterol and vitamin E also help prevent what scientists call clinkers—strange-looking molecules that take up space but are nonfunctional—from entering the cells. These are chemical compounds that contribute to cancer and are prevalent in areas of high pollution.

What does all this mean to the mercury-toxic patient? It means that you should do everything possible to achieve an ideal level of cholesterol to help you overcome the effects of mercury in all of the areas listed above. In studies I performed (and published), I found positive results when people consumed (1) foods in harmony with their ancestral diet, (2) two eggs a day, and (3) up to one-quarter pound of butter a day. In my studies, done twenty years ago, I found that on this diet, high cholesterol levels came down, low cholesterol levels came up, and they stabilized at around 221 milligrams per 100 milliliters of blood. Emmanuel Cheraskin, M.D., D.M.D., formerly of the University of Alabama, recommended a level of 225 milligrams thirty years ago. Forty years ago, Dr. Melvin Page established 222 milligrams as the optimum. All of these recommendations seem to agree that the level of cholesterol at which metabolism is most efficient is between 220 and 225 milligrams per 100 milliliters of blood. Heavy exercise, emotional stress, and medication such as aspirin and other salycilates can artificially lower cholesterol levels, so these should also be avoided.

On the other hand, you don't want to have an artificially elevated level of cholesterol either. So, again, sugar, alcohol, and caffeine should be eliminated. However, many people find that removing sugar, alcohol, and caffeine from their diet is too severe. To make it easier, I recommend switching to honey as a substitute for sugar, decaffeinated beverages or herbal teas as substitutes for caffeine-containing drinks, and nonalcoholic beers and wines to satisfy the psyche's fermentable desires in life. When this has been accomplished, two eggs and up to one-quarter pound of butter daily have been found to be helpful in healing the mercury-toxic patient. Even before my knowledge of mercury toxicity I had my patients on this regimen, and I found that the body optimized its own cholesterol level. Lows were elevated to the ideal level and highs were dropped to the ideal level.

*Triglycerides.* Triglycerides are considered as fats in the blood. They are very large, thick particles that interfere with proper function of the body's chemistry. They cause extra work for the cardiovascular system, and should be kept reasonably low—less than 100 milligrams per 100 milliliters of blood.

Like glucose and cholesterol, triglycerides are elevated by sugar, alcohol, and caffeine, as well as by stress or, as a separate issue, by one's perception of stress. I also see triglycerides elevated in the mercury-toxic patient. Again, getting rid of the amalgam will lower triglycerides, but dietary factors must also be under control at the same time if ideal levels are to be reached.

The most important thing you can do as a mercury-toxic patient to control your triglycerides level is, again, to avoid sugar, alcohol, and caffeine. The next biggest factor in triglyceride elevation is smoking, which causes the body to process heavy metals like mercury ineffectively, and thus slows down the process of healing.

*Total protein and globulin.* In Chapter 6, I discussed the importance of the total protein to globulin (TP/G) ratio in determining the ability of your immune system to fight the effects of mercury toxicity. You know now that vitamin A stimulates the immune system. And you know that mercury can "hit" the immune system, rendering it less effective. Now let's look at the effect of inadequate protein metabolism on your immune system.

There must be sufficient protein in the diet to stimulate the immune system. As is also recommended for those suffering from the condition known as candidiasis, or *Candida albicans,* a very common yeast infection, this protein must be animal protein. For those who are strict vegetarians, I must let you know that your progress may be extremely slow, if you progress at all. I strongly recommend that you discontinue vegetarianism during your treatment period in order to allow the protein fractions in the blood serum to reach a good level. This can be done with eggs and turkey if you prefer to avoid red meats. In nineteen years of treating mercury-toxic patients, I have never been able to help anyone on a vegetarian diet. When people are in good health, they can maintain it on this diet, but for some reason unknown to me they cannot heal from mercury toxicity.

The second thing to realize about protein is that the more it is cooked, the less nutrient is available for your body's use. Beef should be eaten at least medium-rare, and should preferably be grass-fed rather than fattened in a feedlot. Wild game, like venison, is an excellent source of protein.

When the proteins you eat are completely metabolized, amino acids are the resultant product. These are the building blocks from which new protein is assembled to rebuild the body's tissues. If this digestive process is interfered with along the way, uric acid is produced instead of amino acids. My purpose here is to help you do those things that give you an ideal level of globulin and albumin, otherwise known collectively as the total protein.

One easy way to improve protein metabolism is to decrease the amount of liquids you consume with meals to no more than four ounces during the meal, and none for thirty minutes prior to or after the meal. Why are liquids so important in protein metabolism? Go back for a moment to your high school chemistry class. Do you remember that when you studied chemical reactions, you found that anything that diluted the reaction slowed it down? This is what happens with the breakdown of protein in the stomach. In order to begin the breakdown of protein, you must have a sufficient supply of hydrochloric acid (HCl). If you have diluted this acid, as well as the digestive enzymes, with water prior to or during the meal, then it is no longer strong enough to efficiently initiate the beginning steps of metabolism. Therefore, larger protein particles must go into the steps that come next. Because the initial breakdown is inefficient, the whole system suffers. (This increase in the number of larger proteins is one of the causes of allergies.)

You must also make certain that you have sufficient HCl to begin with, and this is where table salt comes into the health picture. The Cl from NaCl (sodium chloride, table salt) is used by the parietal cells in the stomach to produce HCl. Patients on low-salt diets are restricting their ability to metabolize protein. Though it is slightly off the subject at hand, I have never seen an elevated sodium level that was the result of consuming table salt. It may come from sodium preservatives such as those found in soft drinks and margarine (sodium benzoate) and in processed foods (sodium nitrates). It can also be caused by water softeners, mono-sodium glutamate (MSG), and aspirin. So if you have sugar, alcohol, and caffeine out of your diet, you do not need to be worried about table salt.

Let's talk just a moment about milk in protein metabo-lism. This is a problem for children as well as for adults. Milk is chemically classified as a base that neutralizes acid. As a liquid consumed at meals, it not only dilutes the HCl, but it also neutralizes it. The stomach was designed to be efficient at a very low pH, which means a very high acid content. Milk changes this pH so that it is less acidic and, in this way, blocks the absorption of magnesium and calcium in the stomach. This is one of the reasons why milk causes so many allergies. An allergy is a response of the immune system to any "foreign-looking" particle. Large protein particles that were not broken down properly in the stomach are such foreign objects and are called aller-gens. Caffeine and alcohol are also contributors to upset-ting the pH balance. Decaffeinated coffee avoids the caf-feine, but still has the diluting effect.

Albumin is the fraction of the total protein that enables nutrients to be transported through the bloodstream so that they can be made available to the cells. If albumin is low, it does not matter what quality of foods you have eaten. There is no more nutrient available from good foods than from poor ones if sufficient albumin is not there to transport them. Again, decreased fluids during mealtime, increased intake of proteins, and use of digestive enzymes will help.

As a mercury-toxic patient, what are your primary objectives with respect to protein metabolism? Avoid liquid in excess of four ounces at mealtime and use diges-tive enzymes (the ones I use are called Eater's Digest and ProTabs) if the results of your serum protein metabolism tests are either higher or lower than the ideal level. Elimi-nate milk, alcohol, and caffeine as liquids with meals as much as is practical. Make certain there is enough salt in your diet to allow sufficient HCl production. Interestingly enough, the body's hunger sense will tell you when you've had enough salt. After all, nobody sits down and eats cups of salt. The main point is that you don't need to be overly concerned about oversalting your food as long as you use your taste as a guide. Your body was put together with a remarkable ability to determine its needs (as long as additive substances like sugar, alcohol, and caffeine are removed from your diet). Finally, make certain that your protein is not overcooked. Beef should be eaten as rare as possible. Turkey, of course, should be fully cooked, but not cremated. At this time, I do not recommend pork as a source of protein because of its detrimental effect on red blood cells (see Chapter 6). Neither do I recommend fish or shellfish for the mercury-toxic patient. This includes both saltwater and freshwater fish. They are heavily contaminated with methyl mercury, and can slow down the excretion of mercury.

*Lactic dehydrogenase and alkaline phosphatase.* Lactic dehydrogenase (LDH) and alkaline phosphatase (alk phos) are considered liver enzymes. Liver function is the body's last line of defense. If the liver malfunctions, amino acid and vitamin levels in the body drop because they aren't being synthesized, and the levels of LDH and alk phos in the blood rise. There are also some dietary factors that can elevate these two liver enzymes. Alcohol is notable for this.

The foremost cause of an elevated LDH is sugar, because the end result of sugar metabolism is lactic acid, which this enzyme breaks down. The more lactic acid is in your system, the more LDH will be produced to break it down. It can also be elevated by hard cheese and alcohol. The primary way to control LDH is to eliminate sugar, and to supplement your diet with magnesium in an active form (not ground up rocks such as dolomite).

From the standpoint of mercury toxicity, these two enzymes take on a lot more importance. Yes, these enzymes are found in the liver, and liver damage lets them seep out, but, strictly by accident, I found out that there is a lot of both enzymes in red blood cells. Another accidental discovery taught me that as fillings are removed, red blood cells that contain mercury are thrown into the body's recycling bin and dismantled. Heme from hemoglobin, certain amino acids, and other odd parts are reclaimed from the old red cells for remanufacture into new red blood cells. The LDH and alk phos, however, are released into the bloodstream.

Here was born another indicator. When amalgams are removed sequentially and replaced with compatible materials, red cells undergo a rapid degeneration of contaminated cells, together with a regeneration of new red cells. If the treatment is done properly, there will be a decline in red blood cells, hemoglobin, and hematocrit and a simultaneous increase in LDH and alk phos. As the red cells are replenished, the cell figures move toward their optimum levels, and the LDH and alk phos drop to more acceptable levels. It is a measurable scenario.

## Seven Trace Minerals

Let's look now at minerals (as seen in the hair analysis) whose activity is affected by mercury in the system. When looking at mineral levels on the first analysis, I can't be certain whether they are biologically active or not. If the level is in excess of the ideal level, I know that at least some of it is inactive. Years of monitoring thousands of hair reports in conjunction with blood chemistries suggest that the presence of biologically inactive materials shows up as excessive amounts of minerals and a low level usually just means a deficiency. Normally, comparison with the follow-up test (made in about three or four months) will help me determine activity more accurately. I will discuss here only those minerals directly affected by mercury, and what you can do to help your treatment progress more rapidly.

*Calcium.* Remember the calcium-manganese-mercury triad described in our discussion of hair analysis? The most difficult combination to correct includes high calcium. High calcium, by my definition, is calcium exceeding 10 milligrams per 100 milliliters of blood serum, and calcium as seen in hair analysis exceeding 1,000 parts per million in males, or 1,500 parts per million in females. (Low levels of calcium are anything below 9.2 milligrams in the serum and below 300 parts per million in the hair in males, 500 parts per million in females.) There are several ways this can be worsened nutritionally. The number-one dietary cause of elevated calcium is hard cheese. The second is milk and milk products (except butter). Third is the myriad of calcium supplements found on the shelves of drugstores and health food stores. Bone meal and dolomite are two of the worst offenders. But nearly any supplement made of oyster shells or ground-up rocks will do the same thing.

Many people are concerned about osteoporosis and take these calcium supplements in an effort to prevent it. However, I have observed in my patients that bone metabolism (specifically bone density) is controlled by the minerals magnesium and manganese. Inactive forms of calcium serve to interfere with the absorption of the active forms of calcium, magnesium, and manganese. In looking at patient chemistries, I have noted that without the interference of this inactive calcium, over 90 percent of my patients are able to absorb sufficient quantities of active calcium from the foods they eat. Though not a dietary source, hard water can also adversely affect the calcium level. If the water supply is hard where you live, I recommend the use of bottled water.

Why is it so important to avoid an elevated calcium level? Remember that elevated mineral levels indicate the presence of inactive forms of that mineral. Biologically inactive calcium blocks the absorption and the action of active forms of calcium, magnesium, zinc, copper, iron, and manganese. These minerals are extremely important in the system. A too-high level of calcium has also been related to cancer because it adheres to the outside of the cell membrane and causes interference with many other nutrients in their efforts to get into and out of cells as they should.

Calcium is involved in the transmission of nerve impulses. Inactive calcium blocks and inactivates this impulse transmission; it can act as an anesthetic to dull nerve impulses. This is one reason why taking calcium, even when you have too much in your system already, can stop menstrual and leg muscle cramps. It has actually inactivated the transmission of those nerve impulses. But it has not solved the problem that caused the cramps, which is usually a deficiency of magnesium and manganese.

Calcium is highly influential in cell membrane metabolism. Active forms of minerals act like the key to the ignition in an automobile. Inactive forms may move in and take up the same place, but cannot activate chemical reactions. Because they don't have a proper fit, and cannot drive those systems, they cause imbalances. They can block thousands of enzyme systems at any given time.

Because both calcium and magnesium activate the process that begins the production of energy, and because calcium is necessary for the absorption of magnesium, it is easy to understand that the proper amount of biologically active calcium at the cellular level is necessary for you to have a good energy level. Whether you have a deficiency of calcium or you have a contamination of inactive material because of having too much calcium makes no difference as far as the interference with this energy production. The negative result is still the same.

What about deficient calcium? This can be caused by diuretics (water pills and medications such as those given for high blood pressure) and by lecithin (usually from lecithin supplements). It can also be caused by the loss of electrolytes through sweating, whether due to heavy exercise or hot climates.

*Manganese.* The interruption of manganese metabolism is the most consistent disturbance found in patients with periodontal disease, arthritis, MS, muscular dystrophy, cancer, heart disease, and suicidal tendencies. Because of the consistent appearance of manganese deficiency in all degenerative disease, I consider it to be the most important factor in the degenerative disease profile. The action of manganese is blocked first by mercury, and next by calcium. When both factors are present, you have a doubled susceptibility to degenerative disease. Further, continual dietary insults to the body affect the endocrine system, and when these imbalances become greater than what the body can deal with, disease results.

Among other things, manganese:

- Helps to control the glucose level.
- Aids in the calcification of teeth.
- Works with magnesium to prevent muscle cramping.
- Aids in the development of the inner and outer ear.

- Works with magnesium in the control of hyperkinetic and autistic behavior in children.
- Aids in nerve impulse transmission.
- Helps prevent tingling and numbness in the limbs.
- Works with zinc in the prevention of birth defects.

One of the biggest dietary factors that aggravates a manganese deficiency is alcohol, which acts as a diuretic and causes manganese to be excreted in the urine. There are not many causes of an elevated manganese level, but dietary black teas and carrot juice can create some really distinct elevations. According to my studies, an elevation shows up in the hair analysis as anything over 1.2 parts per million; deficiencies as anything under 0.4 parts per million. Carrot juice can cause an increase of several hundred percent, but again, the biological result is too much total manganese with too little of the active form.

Once you lack sufficient manganese, your genetic heritage determines what disease you get. Some of the symptoms of manganese deficiency can be gathered from the list above. They may sound familiar to you by now, as you have already seen them in the list of symptoms of mercury toxicity.

*Mercury.* Although amalgams are the biggest source of exposure to mercury, they are not the only source. You can also ingest large amounts of mercury through your diet (see the lists on pages 153–156 and in Chapter 8).

Probably the greatest dietary source of mercury is tuna. This is followed closely by shellfish like lobster and shrimp. As a rule, the larger the fish, the greater the amount of mercury it contains; however, the scavengers (bottom feeders like catfish, lobsters, or oysters—most shellfish are considered bottom feeders) run a close second. What makes this worse is that this is all in the methyl mercury form. Mercury is methylated by bacteria and floats up into the ocean plankton. Small fish eat the plankton and are in turn eaten by larger fish. Because the fish do not excrete very much methyl mercury (only one percent of what they consume per day), the higher up the food chain you go, the larger the concentrations of methyl mercury. As you have probably realized by now, *any* amount of mercury in the diet can be considered too much.

*Zinc.* Zinc is essential in the activation of over 80 percent of the body's enzyme systems. Perhaps one of its most important functions is in helping to control glucose levels. As mentioned before, zinc is an element in the insulin molecule, which is the control module for glucose. It is also important in the growth of bone, and, along with magnesium, is vital in the healing process. Zinc is critical in the development of all five senses, so it is very important in the development of children. Keep this in mind during pregnancy if your dentist wants to place an amalgam. Mercury, by deactivating zinc, can contribute to birth defects.

Another extremely important function of zinc is the maintenance of healthy skin. Up to 20 percent of the zinc in the body is stored in the skin. When I see a patient with acne, I think first of zinc and those things that block its action, such as inactive calcium and mercury.

Zinc is also necessary for proper sexual function. This is one reason why, when there is a lack of zinc (critical for proper fetal development), there is reduced sex drive, in both males and females. This lack of interest or inability to participate in sexual intercourse may be one of Mother Nature's ways of preventing birth defects that can lead to a deformed child. Zinc also helps to activate the hormones. Perhaps the interference with zinc and manganese activity is part of the reason why methyl mercury toxicity is so damaging genetically (100 times worse than colchicine, widely considered to be the most damaging drug).

Zinc is also necessary in protein metabolism, as well as in the control of post-surgical pain. But the primary function of zinc is the selective alteration of the permeability of the cell membrane. Cells have many pores through which nutrients can enter. Zinc acts as a kind of drawstring that can narrow or widen these pores. Pores that are too small (because of an excess of zinc) keep necessary nutrients from entering; pores that are widened (because of zinc deficiency) may let unnecessary nutrients slip in. The resulting nutritional deficiencies, or excesses, in a cell can cause that cell to die.

Low levels of zinc can be caused by the consumption of caffeine and alcohol, while contamination levels of this mineral are caused by consumption of excess cheese and by supplementation with inactive forms of the mineral. Zinc levels are determined more from hair analysis than from blood chemistry. In both males and females, zinc levels above 220 parts per million are considered high, and levels below 160 parts per million are considered low.

In your diet then, you should avoid hard cheese if your zinc level is elevated. You should avoid sugar, alcohol, and caffeine if your zinc level is deficient, as is seen in so many mercury-toxic patients.

*Magnesium.* The magnesium level is usually taken as a percentage of the calcium level, not as a level in itself. The proper magnesium level is determined by taking the calcium level and dividing it by 7.5. The proper level of magnesium must always be related to the amount of calcium present at that time. A deficiency of magnesium can be caused by alcohol, by birth control pills, and by excess sugar consumption. On the other hand, contamination levels of (inactive) magnesium occur if there is a calcium contamination, or if dolomite is being used as a supplement. Magnesium is involved in the activation of 78 percent of all the enzyme systems. Where there is a lack of magnesium, there is also a higher potential for tooth decay, so as a means of controlling dental problems, magnesium is essential.

Alcohol lowers magnesium levels because it has a diuretic effect. It alters kidney function in such a manner that neither magnesium nor zinc is reclaimed adequately from the urine and sent back to the blood as it should be. Instead, both are excreted.

What must you do to avoid problems with magnesium metabolism? If you have a low magnesium level, you should avoid sugar, alcohol, and caffeine. If you have an elevated magnesium level, you should avoid milk, cheese, and supplements like dolomite and bone meal.

*Chromium.* Chromium levels are identified in the hair analysis. High levels are anything over 1.0 part per million, and low levels are anything under 0.5 parts per million. Low levels of chromium are found in patients who habitually eat large amounts of carbohydrates, have high levels of manganese, or who have contamination levels of vanadium. Vanadium contamination can come from eating chocolate.

A high intake of carbohydrates will lower chromium levels because chromium is necessary in the activation of insulin and is part of what is known as the glucose tolerance factor. This works on cell membranes to allow glucose to get into cells. High levels of carbohydrates, especially sugar, increase the glucose level so that greater amounts of chromium are needed to metabolize it. Most people do not get sufficient amounts of chromium from the foods they eat; this, together with excess demand from a high-carbohydrate diet, contributes to many cases of deficiency. I find that when a patient has a low chromium level, it is difficult to control his or her glucose level. Therefore it is necessary to be very strict about dietary control and taking supplementation.

*Potassium.* Potassium levels, as seen in the blood chemistry, are deemed high if they are over 4.8 milligrams per 100 milliliters of serum; low levels are anything under 4.2 milligrams. In the hair analysis, amounts below 35 parts per million are deficient, and amounts above 65 parts per million are excessive. Low levels of potassium can be caused by drugs such as cortisone, blood pressure medications (diuretics), and birth control pills. Nearly all medications and drugs will upset potassium metabolism. Alcohol and exercise can also cause potassium deficiencies. High levels (again, representing an excess of the inactive, nonbiological form) are found when a patient uses "lite" salt, kelp, or sea salt. Lite salt is potassium chloride (KCl). This is especially bad when it comes to upsetting the fluid balance, because it upsets the ratio between sodium and potassium. Fluid balance is the difference in the amount of fluid inside the cell versus the amount outside the cell. Obviously, our fluids (such as water) come from outside the body. They are absorbed through the intestinal tract, transported to the cells, and if cell membranes are in good shape, they allow the right amount of water in. If a cell does not bring in *enough* water, then the concentrations of chemicals inside become too high, which destroys the cell. If a cell brings in *too much* water, then the concentration of water is too high, which dilutes the cell. By causing cells to burn up or to become waterlogged, lite salt leads to cell death either way. Kelp and sea salt have also been noted to upset this ratio to a lesser extent.

Potassium deficiency and/or contamination is characteristic of MS patients, and is the number-two deficiency in the periodontal patient. A proper balance between potassium and sodium is extremely important, and extremely difficult to achieve. It takes a long time to build up healthy levels of sodium and potassium. I have noted that levels of these two minerals can drop even if they initially appear to be within body chemistry ideals, because it is so easy to get contamination from inactive sources. The first hair analysis I do on a patient very seldom shows an abundance of active minerals.

### Foods to Eat and Foods to Avoid

In addition to improving nutrition by monitoring the body's level of minerals and trace elements, the mercury-toxic patient should follow a number of simple guidelines in choosing which foods to eat. The following are some of the most important foods to eat for a mercury-free diet, and what they do for your body.

*Beef, turkey, chicken.* These three are the most familiar and readily available primary protein sources. Wild game like venison, antelope, and elk—though harder to get hold of—are quite good. Here in the Midwest, we can even get buffalo. Game fowl like wild turkey, duck, quail, and goose are good also. Basically, most animal sources (with the exception of fish and pork) are reasonably decent. All these foods supply protein, which stabilizes glucose levels; bolsters the immune system; and provides amino acids, which serve as the building blocks for growth and repair.

*Butter.* Butter optimizes cholesterol levels and enhances absorption of nutrients.

*Eggs.* Eggs optimize cholesterol levels and provide protein.

*Salt*. Salt aids in protein metabolism and aids in the transport of nutrients through cell membranes.

Now, let's outline once again those things that should be *avoided* if you are suffering from mercury toxicity, and the reasons why.

*Alcohol*. Alcohol raises serum glucose, cholesterol, triglycerides, alk phos, and LDH; upsets the endocrine balance; depletes magnesium, zinc, manganese, potassium, and folic acid (which is also knocked out by mercury); and interferes with protein metabolism if taken at mealtime.

*Caffeine*. Caffeine raises serum glucose, cholesterol, triglycerides, and uric acid; upsets the endocrine balance; interferes with protein metabolism; and depletes magnesium, zinc, and chromium.

*Cheese*. Cheese raises LDH and other liver function tests, and elevates the levels of nonbiological forms of calcium, magnesium, and zinc.

*Chocolate*. Chocolate raises serum glucose, cholesterol, triglycerides, and uric acid; upsets the endocrine balance; interferes with protein metabolism; and depletes magnesium, zinc, and chromium.

*Fish and seafood*. Fish (including tuna) and seafood contain methyl mercury.

*Inactivate supplements*. The most common inactivate supplements are the calcium-magnesium compounds, specifically dolomite, bone meal, and oyster shell. If oyster shells were really soluble, they would dissolve in the ocean! The others are also in nonbiological forms, meaning that they are not connected with any protein or enzyme that would allow them to be properly processed in the body. If you *put* it into your body, your body has to do something with it, and it usually ends up taking up space where normal metabolism would otherwise occur. This is what is meant by *contamination*. When you get the contamination (or nonbiological) form of a supplement, it usually does more harm than good, because it prevents normal metabolism from taking place.

**Liquids with meals.** Drinking liquids with meals interferes with protein metabolism.

**Lite salt.** Lite salt products elevate potassium levels.

**Margarine.** Margine contains cadmium, which blocks the action of zinc. It also contains sodium preservatives, which upset the sodium balance.

**Milk.** Milk raises the level of nonbiological calcium and interferes with protein metabolism.

**Refined carbohydrates.** Sugar is the most common form of refined carbohydrate. Literally thousands of other foods contain sugar as well. White flour is another common refined carbohydrate, and the combination of white flour *and* sugar, of course, is found in most bakery goods, breakfast cereals, and other popular products. Refined carbohydrates raise serum glucose, cholesterol, and triglycerides; upset the endocrine balance; and deplete chromium and manganese.

**Smoking.** Tobacco is not a food, of course, but it has a negative effect on the entire body chemistry. It raises cholesterol and triglycerides; raises lead and nickel levels;

and interferes with cell membrane metabolism, which slows the excretion of mercury.

*Soft drinks.* Soft drinks contain sugar, caffeine, sodium preservatives, and sodium-containing artificial sweeteners.

*Sugar.* Sugar raises serum glucose, cholesterol, and triglycerides; upsets the endocrine balance; and depletes chromium, zinc, magnesium, and manganese.

As you can see by now—if you hadn't before—it is easier to place a filling than it is to trace its devastating biological domino effect. And as complex and far-reaching as these areas are, they represent only a fraction of the total effect. Most of the problems take place at the cellular and even the molecular level, and only become visible as changes in blood chemistry after the function of *billions* of cells has been altered.

# 8

# Other Sources of Mercury Exposure

*A*malgam is not the only source of mercury exposure. However, mercury toxicity cannot be treated successfully until *all* amalgam is out of the mouth.

During the initial treatment phase, it is important to avoid exposure to other sources of mercury. In this chapter I will list as many sources of exposure as I know of at the current time. Most of them can be avoided quite easily. After initial treatment is completed and you are on a maintenance regimen, you may find that occasional exposure does not affect you severely. Just remember, though, that once you have been sensitized to something like mercury, you can always expect to have some type of reaction to any future exposure.

There are dozens of lists in both scientific and lay literature of potential sources of mercury. One book claims that there are over 4,000 commercial uses of mercury. I don't remember where I read that, but I remember the feeling of hopelessness I experienced knowing that I could list fewer than 100. Here is a list that will give you an idea of relatively common things you should consider avoiding. (I have noticed that some manufacturers have reduced the mercury content or even discontinued some products since general awareness of the problem has risen. These changes have been made because people like you have questioned the manufacturers.)

Some of the most common exposures to mercury come through foods, cosmetics, medications, household chemicals, gardening chemicals, and other items that contain high levels of mercury, as well as professions and industries in which people are exposed to mercury.

## FOODS

In addition to the foods mentioned in Chapter 7, the following should be avoided:

- Grains treated with methyl mercury fungicides, especially wheat.
- Kelp and other seaweeds.
- Large saltwater fish like swordfish, salmon, cod, etc.
- Shellfish, including shrimp, lobster, crab, oyster, etc.
- Tuna, canned or fresh.

## COSMETICS

Some cosmetics are also high in mercury, including:

- Some hair dyes.
- Mascara, especially waterproof.

• Skin-lightening creams.

## MEDICATIONS

Your medicine cabinet may also contain high-mercury items. Here is a list of some of them, broken down into different categories:

### Antiseptic and First-Aid Preparations

• AAA Paste
• Acid Jelly and Benzo-caine
• Bag Balm
• Calamine Lotion
• Calomel (powder and talc)
• Dermacol liquid
• Dermato ointment
• Hermesol
• I.P.S. ointment
• Kay-Sen
• Lanacane
• Lubafax
• Marsa
• Massengill's Tannic Acid Jelly and Benzocaine
• Mazon
• Mercoseptic
• Mercurochrome
• Merthiolate
• Mertok
• Metaphen
• Mycolog cream
• Mystacin cream
• Palmer's Antiseptic Lotion
• Pheocol paste
• Phillips Corona ointment
• Pike's Lotion
• Prosol
• Pureapas Blue ointment
• Raleigh's ointment
• Rexall Skin Antiseptic
• Sperti ointment
• T.R. ointment
• Thimerosal
• TPA ointment

- Unguentine
- Verthal

- Zemacol

## Psoriasis Preparations

- Ammoniated mercury
- Ar-Ex Sorsis creams
- Dermoil
- Dural Cade Oil Cream
- Psoriasis Treatment Lotion

- Riasol lotion
- Siroil
- Soridex
- Unguentum Bossi

## Fungicides

- Amber Liquid
- Athlete Ointment
- Epidex
- Gebauer's PMC Spray

- Maseda Foot Powder
- Melsan
- Phe-Mer-Nite
- Phytox-Ointment

## Acne Preparations

- Derma-Teen Skin Soap
- Derma-Tone

- Dermathyer Cream
- Teen-Ac

## Bleaching Creams

- Blue Ointment
- Brightener
- Esoterica Medicated Face Cream
- Golden Peacock Bleach Cream
- JA-GO-DA Face Cream

- Madam C.J. Walker Skin Cream
- Mercolized Cream
- Natinola Bleach Cream
- Peacock's Imperial Cream
- Stillman's Freckle Cream

## Eye Preparations

- Allerest Eye Drops
- Blinx Eye Wash liquid
- Clean-N-Soak
- Collyrium lotion
- Coloptin
- Contact lens solutions
- Dr. Petit's American Eye Salve
- Eyelo-Drop
- Murine
- Nozmol
- Prefrin-Z Liquifilm
- Smooth Eye decongestant
- Wetting solution
- Yellow mercuric oxide ointment

## Ear Preparations

- Otall Ear Drops

## Nasal Preparations (Drops and Spray)

- Afrin
- Clopane
- Neo-Synephrine
- Neotrol
- Privine
- Saline nose drops
- Vasefrin
- Vasohist

## Throat Lozenges

- B & R Homeopathic Tablets No. 195A
- Phe-Mer-Caine
- Phe-Mer-Nite
- Thantis

## Hemorrhoidal Ointments and Suppositories

- Kip Hemorrhoid Relief Ointment
- Lanacane cream
- Preparation H

### Vaginal Jellies, Tablets, and Douches

- Baculin
- Dorana
- Koromex
- Lorophyn
- Merpertogel
- Neovagisal
- Norforms

- Nylmerate II Solution Concentrate
- Phe-Mer-Nite
- Servex
- Southern Pharmacal
- Tricho-San
- Triserts
- Vagisil

### Hair Tonic (Mercuric Chloride)

- Bar soap
- Elm's Hair and Soap Treatment

- Scalpo ointment

### Veterinary Preparations

- Bag Balm
- Dr. Daniel's Gall Salve, Hoof Ointment and Softener

- McClellan's Eyelid Ointment
- Mulrilicare
- Stevens Ointment

### Prophylactic Kits

- Dough-Boy

## HOUSEHOLD CHEMICALS

Beware of chemicals used for household repairs and hobbies, such as:

- Yellow, vermillion, and cinnabar pigments of paints, dyes, and inks, like Weber vermillion.

- Mildew- and corrosion-resistant paints (phenylmercuric compounds), like Bay State One-Coat Mildew Resistant White.
- Mildew preventatives, like Fen and Mer-Q-Ree.
- Anti-fouling paint for boats (mercuric oxides), like Federal Anti-Fouling Paint.
- Wood preservatives (ethyl mercury chloride).
- Photographic solutions.
- Gun bluing.
- Tile cement.
- Lead mercury solder.
- Many latex and oil-based paints.

## GARDENING CHEMICALS

Even your lawn and garden are suspect. Below are some items to avoid using.

### Seed Fungicides, Protectants, and Disinfectants

- Amacene
- Gallotox
- Gy-Treet SQS
- Isotox Seed Treater
- Merc-O-Dent
- Mergama "C"
- Merlane liquid
- Merlane dust
- Panodrin
- Panogen
- Pantirra
- Parson's Seed Saver dust
- Semesan

### Turf Fungicides and Disinfectants

- Calocine
- Caloclor
- Calogreen
- Coromerc

- Corrosive Sublimate
- Mersolite-8
- Mersolite-90

- PHIX
- PM Grain Protectant
- Semesay

### Plant Fungicides
- Orchard Brand Mercury Spray
- Puratized Apple Spray

- Puratized Agricultural Spray
- Semesan fungicide

### Herbicides
- Blitz
- Dynaside Homelawn Crabgrass

- Killer
- PMAS
- Puraturf

### Insecticides
- Green Cross
- Hubbard Cabbage Maggot Dust
- Magic Brand Bug Killer
- Mergamma
- P & P Cabbage Maggot

- Real-Kill Bug Killer Destroyer
- Real-Kill Moth Bomb
- Setrete
- Setrete mist

### MISCELLANEOUS

Here are some miscellaneous items to beware of:

- Adhesives
- Air conditioner filters
- Batteries with mercury cells
- Cinnabar, used in jewelry

- Fabric softeners
- Felts
- Floor waxes and polishes
- Sewage disposal
- Tattoos

## PROFESSIONS

You can find mercury in your professional world, too:

- For barbers and hairdressers: disinfectants like MEMA, Pomerio 18, and Germicides (phenylmercuric iodide and nitrate).
- For laboratory workers: mercurial reagents.
- For physicians, laboratory workers, and morticians: tissue fixatives like Helly's and Zember's.
- For dentists and dental technicians: dental amalgams.
- For nurses: mercurial diuretics like dicurin procaine, mercubydoin, and thiomerin sodium.

## INDUSTRIAL PROCESSES

There are numerous industries in which workers can be exposed to mercury. Some of the most mercury-toxic processes in the working world include:

- Alloy handling with tin and copper
- Artificial silk manufacturing
- Bactericide production
- Barometer manufacturing
- Battery manufacturing
- Bronzing
- Calibration instrument manufacturing
- Cap loading, percussion
- Carbon brush making
- Caustic soda production
- Chlorine production
- Dentistry
- Direct current meter manufacturing
- Disinfectant production
- Drug manufacturing
- Dye manufacturing
- Electric apparatus manufacturing
- Electrode manufacturing
- Electroplating
- Embalming

- Explosives production
- Farming
- Felt manufacturing
- Fingerprint detecting
- Fireworks manufacturing
- Fish cannery work
- Fungicide production
- Fur preservation
- Fur processing
- Gold extracting
- Histology
- Ink making
- Insecticide production
- Investment casing workers
- Jewelry production and repair
- Laboratory work (chemical)
- Lampmaking (fluorescent)
- Lead-mercury soldering
- Manometer manufacturing
- Mercury pump manufacturing
- Mercury refining
- Mining, mercury
- Mining, gold
- Mirror production
- Neon light manufacturing
- Paint manufacturing
- Printing
- Papermaking
- Pesticide production and application
- Photography
- Pressure gauge manufacturing
- Seed handling
- Silver extracting
- Steel etching
- Switch making
- Tannery work
- Taxidermy
- Textile printing
- Thermometer making
- Vinyl chloride manufacturing
- Working with mercury

You can see how many places mercury is used in our modern environment. It is impossible to avoid all sources, but you should make every reasonable effort you can. Read labels carefully, and question every product mentioned in the list. There are usually acceptable substitutes for any product. For example, makers of contact lens solutions know that some people are allergic to the thimerosal preservative (a mercury compound) used in their products. So there is at least one solution of every type (cleaning, soaking, etc.) for both hard and soft lenses that is preservative-free. Check with your ophthalmologist if you need these solutions.

Now for the good news—and the bad news. After your amalgams are out and your body is cleaned up and recovered, a new protective mechanism takes over. This is called the secondary immune response. During the first three to six months after removal (provided you behave yourself), your immune system will recover and start listening to "memory cells." These are white blood cells that "remember the Alamo," so to speak, and sound the alarm at the slightest hint of mercury invasion. This is an excellent aid to help you avoid further exposure, but it can seem like a real negative at times.

For instance, you are at a fine restaurant and have their special of the day. Ever notice that dinner specials are almost always fish? They are. So you enjoy a meal of the finest fish in town, then your memory cells sound the alarm. Diarrhea, vomiting, tears, and increased excretion of ear wax hit simultaneously in about forty-five minutes. Let's see you act graciously and try to find a restroom while everyone else is eating dessert.

These reactions do teach you the value of avoidance, but they often require a change in lifestyle and trifocals to read the labels. Of course, if you want to tough out the exposure, you can. We all have our own ways of learning.

# 9
# Follow-Up Testing and Lifestyle

*A*fter the diagnosis is made and the treatment plan initiated, then what happens? It's like shooting at a target over the hill. How do you know if you hit the target? That's what follow-up testing is all about. Of course, the alleviation of symptoms is the bottom line for you personally. You want to have more energy, stop having seizures, and feel good about life instead of being depressed. But you also need scientific proof, or you too may decide it was "all in your head."

## FOLLOW-UP PROCEDURES

As I have mentioned, blood profile, CBC, hair analysis, and urinary excretion are the basic tests used to determine the extent of mercury toxicity. If progress is being made, these chemistries should change for the better.

Diagnosis is based on these tests, but from the research done in eighteen other areas, I know these are not all the changes that take place following amalgam removal. The four basics provide an affordable analysis that covers the major areas of imbalance, but not every imbalance. If some other external factor is at fault, then the basic chemistries are not likely to respond. Fortunately, chemistries that don't respond usually point toward the area of interference, and from that I can figure out where to look next.

For the most part, following up with a repeat of three of the four initial tests gives a good overview of a patient's progress. The CBC, blood profile, and urine mercury excretion tests can show significant changes in anywhere from a few days to three weeks. From these tests, I can get a good, quick, inexpensive indication of progress. At the present time, I look at follow-up tests on my patients three weeks after amalgam removal has been completed, then three months, and then every six months.

I look first at urinary excretion of mercury. If the excretion level has not risen, I do not expect much change in the other chemistries. This is the time to reassess the original chemistries and the diet to see if something was overlooked, or if the patient is really following the dietary recommendations and avoiding other exposures. The most common problem I find is that the patient is still consuming caffeine or eating fish. Also, since the supplementation plan is originally designed as conservatively as possible, the patient may not be taking enough of a particular supplement to activate the mercury excretion mechanism. If that is the case, the supplementation regimen is then altered to meet the patient's needs.

Next, I look at the CBC. Since fatigue is a major factor in so many people, hemoglobin and hematocrit levels are of primary concern. They may improve by going *either* up or down. That sounds illogical until you think again about the chemistry. If hemoglobin is saturated with mercury, it is not transporting oxygen. The body's compensatory mechanism is to produce high amounts of red cells, yet because of the mercury, all these new cells cannot do their job and the symptom is fatigue. When enough mercury is removed to allow the production of mercury-free red blood cells, then the red cell count goes down because a greater amount of oxygen is being transported in the available cells.

White blood cells are a prime factor in people whose immune systems are not up to par. At three weeks after amalgam removal, several up-and-down swings have usually taken place, and a pseudostability may have occurred. Dozens of changes can happen here for each individual type of white cell. Each of the various combinations of up and down carries a different interpretation. The excitement I feel is high when I follow changes in the white blood cells, because the changes occur rapidly and in direct proportion to the response of the body's immune system. For instance, white blood cells called monocytes appear to clean up the debris (fragments from mercury-compromised cells) left behind by the ravages of mercury toxicity. Monocyte levels that go down indicate that less trash needs to be removed; therefore, progress is being made. Patients enjoy watching the progress of these cells, too, because generally as the number of cleaner-uppers goes down, the health goes up.

Blood serum chemistry is partly mercury-related and partly related to nutrition. It is the most complex area to interpret in follow-up for that reason. All the other chemistries, plus diet and lifestyle, play a role in altering the levels of glucose, cholesterol, triglycerides, and total protein. This doesn't mean that it is impossible to interpret, just that each factor has to be weighed against all the other factors known to produce changes. For the most part, when the body has an opportunity to heal (as it does upon the removal of a toxin like mercury), all systems work together to produce a better, healthier body. This produces predictable changes in the chemistry, and an outlying factor is easy to spot. For instance, glucose, cholesterol, and triglycerides all should respond in like fashion to dietary sins. But if all the sugar, alcohol, and caffeine are removed from the diet, and only the cholesterol and triglycerides respond, then an outlying medical factor—such as diabetes—may be causing some of the trouble. These factors usually require special attention.

How long do you have to remain on a good diet and take supplements? Once your body has been challenged with mercury and lost the battle—once you've gotten sick—you are more susceptible to recurrence than is your neighbor who didn't get sick. The answer could be: As long as you want to be in better health. A good diet is a good idea for anyone. However, while supplementation is often necessary for basic correction, it is not always necessary forever. If you have access to organically grown foods and good water, you may be able to derive all of the nutrients you need from your foods. If your body has sustained some direct blows and needs more of a particular substance than is available in a normal diet, supplementation may be required for many years.

This is where follow-up with both blood and hair analysis comes in. After you have had your amalgams removed, have made alterations in your diet, have avoided excess mercury exposure, and have been on supplementation for four to six months, a repeat hair analysis will let you know what is happening within the cells over an extended period of time. In other words, it will let you know what your new lifestyle is doing for you. It will enable you to further refine your diet and your supplementation based upon your current needs. I personally check my own chemistry about every six months, and I recommend this for all of my patients.

Even without a hair analysis, though, maintenance supplementation can be good preventive medicine. Maintenance dosages will not cause imbalances. Maintenance in my practice usually consists of TransMix, to enhance generalized absorption, and vitamin C. Vitamin C helps condition your cell membranes to allow better selection of nutrients for absorption and more discerning exclusion of potentially harmful substances. It is also the prime initiator of·the basic energy unit called cyclic adenosine monophosphate (CAMP), which is the initial group of chemicals that eventually produces ATP—the basic source of energy for every cell's metabolic activity.

Optional supplementation includes digestive enzymes if the body continues to need help in protein metabolism, and Vitamate for a well-balanced, daily vitamin-mineral combination that does not overdose any area. Vitamate is a vitamin-mineral combination put together in what we call the "matrix." This is a system that allows minerals multiple routes of absorption into the body. By having the vitamins and minerals together in the matrix, we can use very low dosages and achieve very high absorption. This has been a real asset to my practice, because the overdoses frequently seen elsewhere do not develop.

Beyond this, I prefer to be able to monitor and prescribe specific courses of action for your needs on the basis of chemistry excesses and deficiencies. There are a few exceptions, of course. Taking up to 400 international units (IUs) of Vitamin E a day is fine. (Some people react adversely above that figure.) Multiple vitamins are okay, as long as the vitamin B12 does not exceed 10 micrograms daily. More than this amount depletes the body of folic acid, which is one of the primary vitamin deficiencies created by mercury.

## CONCLUSION

I hope you have concluded by now that you don't want mercury in your molars. Granted, there are other dental materials that are bad, but there has to be a starting point to gain the attention of the public, and someday of dentistry.

My hope is that through this book you have gained sufficient understanding and knowledge to help direct your own treatment in getting rid of harmful dental fillings and replacing them with dental materials that are compatible with your immune system.

Remember, please don't harass your own dentist about the mercury issue if he or she shows high resistance. As of this writing, in all states except California, dentists are threatened with the loss of their license to practice if they so much as mention to a patient that mercury might be hazardous. If you run into this problem, please call the Huggins Diagnostic Center for a referral to dentists in your area who have been trained in these techniques. I can at least help you to obtain a blood test for compatible dental materials to avoid experiencing the out-of-the-frying-pan-into-the-fire syndrome.

The Center's telephone number for information is 1–800–331–2303. Good luck!

# References

Anderson, W.A.D. *Synopsis of Pathology*, Fourth Edition. Saint Louis: C.V. Mosby Co., 1957.

Baasch, E. "Theoretical Reflections on the Etiology of Multiple Sclerosis. Is Multiple Sclerosis a Mercury Allergy?" *Schweis Arch. Neuolchir. Psychiat.* 98:1, 1966.

Castle, et al. Mentioned in J.L. Bernier, *The Management of Oral Disease*. Saint Louis: C.V. Mosby Co., 1955.

Collins, N.J. "A Concept of the Etiology of Leukemia." *Bulletin of Cancer Progress*, 9:2 (March-April 1959).

Comroe, B.I., L.H. Collins, and M.P. Crane. *Internal Medicine in Dental Practice*, Fourth Edition. Lea & Febiger.

Cutright, D.E., et al. "Systemic Mercury Levels Caused by Inhaling Mist During High-Speed Amalgam Grinding." *Journal of Oral Medicine*, Vol. 28, No. 4 (October-December 1973).

Eggleston, D.W., and M. Nylander. "Correlation of Dental Amalgam With Mercury in Brain Tissue." *Journal of Prosthetic Dentistry*, 58 (1987).

Eyl, Thomas B. "Methyl Mercury Poisoning in Fish and

Human Beings." *Modern Medicine*, Vol. 38, November 1970.

Gay, D.D., R.D. Cox, and J.W. Reinhard. "Chewing Releases Mercury from Fillings." *Lancet*, 5 May 1979.

Goldberg, M.A. *Materials Used in Dentistry and Their Manipulation*, Fourth Edition. Ann Arbor, MI: The University of Michigan Press, 1949.

Hagar, R.N., S. Schermerhorn, C. Schroeder, and R.H. Reger. "Mercury Hygiene in the Dental Office." *Journal of the Colorado Dental Association*, 54:1 (September 1975).

Hammond, A.L. "Mercury in the Environment: Natural and Human Factors." *Science*, 171:3973 (1971).

Harper, W.E. "Amalgam Failures. Where is the Fault: In the Alloy or in the Operator?" *Dominion Dental Journal*, 40:153 (May 1928).

Heintze, M., et al. "Methylation of Mercury From Dental Amalgam and Mercuric Chloride by Oral Streptococci in Vitro." *Scandinavian Journal of Dental Research*, 9, 1993.

Hepburn, W.B. "Behavior of Metal Dental Fillings in the Mouth." *British Dental Journal*, 33:1131 (1912).

Hernberg, S., and E. Hasanen. "Relation of Inorganic Mercury in Blood and Urine." *Work, Environment, Health*, 8:ISS 2 (1971).

Hollander, L. "Galvanic Burns of Oral Mucosa." *Journal of the American Medical Association*, 99:383 (July 30, 1932).

Hollander, L., H.H. Permar, and L. Shonfield. "Leukoplakia of Oral Mucosa." *Journal of the American Dental Association*, 20:41 (January 1933).

Hyams, B.L. "The Electrogalvanic Compatibility of Orthodontic Materials." *International Journal of Orthodontics and Dentistry for Children*, 19:9 (1933).

Hyams, B.L., and H.C. Ballon. "Dissimilar Metals in Mouths as Possible Cause of Otherwise Unexplainable Symptoms." *Canadian Medical Association Journal*, 28:488 (November 1933).

Lain, E.S., W. Schriever, and G.S. Caughron. "Problem of Electrogalvanism in the Oral Cavity Caused by Dissimilar Metals." *Journal of the Amercian Dental Association*, 27:1765 (November 1940).

Lain, E.S. "Nickel Dermatitis, New Source." *Journal of the American Medical Association*, 96:771 (March 7, 1931).

Lain, E.S. "Chemical and Electrolytic Lesion of the Mouth Caused by Artificial Dentures." *Archives of Dermatology and Syphilis*, 25:21 (1932).

Lain, E.S. "Electrogalvanic Lesions of Oral Cavity Produced by Metallic Dentures." *Journal of the American Medical Association*, 100:717 (March 11, 1933).

Lain, E.S., and G.S. Caughron. "Electrogalvanic Phenomena of Oral Cavity Caused by Dissimilar Metallic Restoration." *Journal of the American Dental Association*, 23:1641 (September 1936).

Lain, E.S., W. Schriever, and G.S. Caughron. "Problem of Electrogalvanism in the Oral Cavity Caused by Dissimilar Metals." *Journal of the American Dental Association*, 1765 (November 1940).

Lane, J.R. "Survey of Dental Alloys." *Journal of the American Dental Association*, 39:414 (October 1949).

Lenhan, J.M., H. Smith, and W. Harvey. "Mercury Hazards in Dental Practice." *British Dental Journal*, 135 (1973).

Leyva, J.C. Alergia del mercurio con dermatitis eczematica causada pro calzas de amalgama de plata. Personal communication, Carrera 10a, 9727, Apt. 302, Bogota, Columbia.

Leyva, J.C. Algunas consideraciones sobre amalgamas dentales. Personal communication.

Leyva, J.C. A case of hypersensitivity (allergy) for mercury. Personal communication.

Leyva, J.C. Exposicion pro um periodo largo de los dentistas al mercurio. Personal communication.

Leyva, J.C. Mercurio-quimica y mecanismo de accion. Personal communication.

Leyva, J.C. Significado para la salud del mercurio usado em pratica dental. Personal communication.

Lindstedt, G. "A Rapid Method for the Determination of Mercury in Urine." *Analyt.*, 95, March 1970.

Lindstedt, G., and I. Skare. "Microdetermination of Mercury in Biological Samples." *Analyt.*, 66, March 1971.

Lippmann, A. "Disorders Caused by Electric Discharges in the Mouth With Artificial Dentures." *Deutsche Med. Wchnschr.*, 56:1394 (1930).

Lu, F.C., P.E. Berteau, and D.J. Clegg. "The Toxicity of Mercury in Man and Animals." Part of Technical Report No. 137, *Mercury Contamination in Man and his Environment*, International Atomic Energy Agency, Vienna, Austria, July 1972.

Manning, P.R. "Electrolytic Theory of Dental Caries." *Pacific Dental Gazette*, 26:365 (June 1918).

Mantyla, D.G., and O.D. Wright. "Mercury Toxicity in the Dental Office: A Neglected Problem." *Journal of the American Dental Association*, 92:6 (June 1976).

Mays, C. "No Battery in a Tooth." *Advertizer*, 12:103 (1880).

McGehee, W.H.C., H.A. True, and F.L. Inskipp. *A Textbook of Operative Dentistry*, Fourth Edition. New York: McGraw-Hill, 1956.

Menkin, V. "Growth-Promoting Factor in Exudates, Mechanism of Repair and Pre-Neoplastic-Like Responses." *Cancer Research*, 17:963-969 (1957).

Meyer, mentioned in Traub and Holmes, *Archives of Dermatology and Syphilis*, 38:349 (1938).

Morrison, M.A. "Electric Currents in Oral Cavity." *Dominion Dental Journal*, 14:86 (January 1902).

Mumford, J.M. "Electrolytic Action in the Mouth and its Relationship to Pain." *Journal of Dental Research*, 636, August 1957.

Nixon, G.S. "Mercury in Dental Surgery." *British Dental Surgical Assistant*, 29:6, 1971,107–109.

Palmer, S.B. "Dental Decay and Filling Materials Considered in Their Electrical Relations." *American Journal of Dental Science*, 12:105 (1878).

Palmer, S.B. "Electrochemical Theory." *American Journal of Dental Science*, 14:166 (1880).

Palmer, S.B. "Electricity in the Mouth." *Dental Items of Interest*, 10:399 (September 1888).

Patrick, J.J.R. "Oral Electricity and the New Departure." *Dental Cosmos*, 22:543 (October 1880).

Pleva, Jaro. "Mercury Poisoning from Dental Amalgam." *Journal of Orthomolecular Psychiatry*, Vol. 12, No. 3 (September 1983).

Polia, J.H. "What the Physicians Should Know About Dental Problems." *Journal of the American Dental Association*, 20:2169 (December 1933).

Radics, J., et al. "Die Kristallinin Komponenten der Silberamalgam Untersuchungen mit der Elektronishchen Rontgenmikrosorde." *Zahnarztl. Welt* 79, 1031, 1970.

Roome, N.W., and A.A. Dahlberg. "Electrochemical Ulcer of Buccal Mucosa (Case Report)." *Journal of the American Dental Association,* 23:1652 (September 1936).

Roper, L.H. "Restorations With Amalgam in the Army: An Evaluation and Analysis." *Journal of the American Dental Association,* 34:443 (April 1, 1947).

Schoonover, I.C., and W. Sounder. "Research on Dental Materials at the National Bureau of Standards." H.B.S., Circular 497 (Washington, D.C.: U.S. Government Printing Office, August 15, 1950).

Schoonover, I.C., W. Sounder, and J.R. Beall. "Excessive Expansion of Dental Amalgam." *Journal of the American Dental Association,* 28:1278 (August 1941).

Schoonover, I.C., and W. Sounder. "Corrosion of Dental Alloys." *Journal of the American Dental Association,* 28, August 1941.

Schoonover, I.C., and W. Sounder. "Corrosion of Dental Alloys." *Journal of the American Dental Association,* 28 (Part 2), 1278, 1941.

Schriever, W., and L.E. Diamond. "Electromotive Forces and Electric Currents Caused by Metallic Dental Fillings." *Journal of Dental Research,* 31:205 (April 1952).

Schriever, W., and L.E. Diamond, "Electromotive Forces and Electric Currents Caused by Metallic Dental Fillings." *Journal of Dental Research,* 18:205 (1938).

Schwisheimer, W. "Mercury Vapors in Dental Offices and Laboratories: Prevention of Poisoning." *Zahntchnik,* 29:4 (1971).

Sharma, R.P., and E.J. Obersteiner. "Metals and Neurotoxic Effects: Cytotoxicity of Selected Metallic Compounds on Chick Ganglia Cultures." *Journal of Comparative Pathology* 91, 235 (1981).

Simon, W.J. *Clinical Operative Dentistry*. Philadelphia: W.B. Saunders Co., 1956.

Smith. "Alloys of Gallium With Powdered Metals as Possible Replacement for Dental Amalgam." *Journal of the American Dental Association*, 53:415-424, 1956.

Sodeman, W.A. *Pathologic Physiology*, Second Edition. Philadelphia: W.B. Saunders Co., 1956.

Solomon, H.A., M.C. Reinhard, and H.I. Goodale. "Precancerous Oral Lesions From Electrical Causes." *The Dental Digest*, 39:142 (1933).

Solomon, H.A., and M.C. Reinhard. "Electric Phenomena From Dental Materials." Dental *Survey*, 9:23 (January 1933).

Solomon, H.A., and M.C. Reinhard. "Inhibitory Factors in Galvanism." *American Journal of Cancer*, 22:606 (November 1934).

Solomon, H.A., and M.C. Reinhard. "Inhibitory Factors in Galvanism From Dental Metals." *Dental Cosmos*, 68:1259 (December 1936).

Solomon, H.A., M.C. Reinhard, and H.L. Goltz. "Salivary Influence on Galvanism." *Dental Items of Interest*, 60:1047 (November 1938).

Solomon, H.A., M.C. Reinhard, and H.I. Goodale. "Precancerous Lesions From Electrical Causes." *Dental Digest*, 39:149 (1933).

Stallard, H., Silver amalgam as a tooth repair material. Personal communication, 275 Altamirano Way, San Diego, California.

Stock. Alfred. "Die Chronish Quecksilber und Amalgam Vergiftung." *Zahnarztl. Rumdschau*, 48, 1939.

Strader, K.H. "Amalgam Alloy: Its Heat Treatment, Flow, Mercury Content and Distribution of Dimensional Change." *Journal of the American Dental Association*, 38:602 (May 1949).

Summers, A.O., J. Wireman, M.J. Vimy, F. L. Lorscheider, B. Marshall, S.B. Levy, S. Bennett, and L. Billard. "Mercury Released from Dental 'Silver' Fillings Provokes an Increase in Mercury- and Antibiotic-Resistant Bacteria in Oral and Intestinal Floras of Primates." *Antimicrobial Agents and Chemotherapy*, April 1993.

Svare, C.W., et al. "The Effect of Dental Amalgams on Mercury Levels in Expired Air." *Journal of Dental Research* 50 (September 1981).

Sweeney, J.T. "Manipulation of Amalgam to Prevent Excess Distortion and Corrosion. *Journal of the American Dental Association*, 31:375 (March 1944).

Trakhtenberg, I.M. *Chronic Effects of Mercury on Organisms*. Department of Health, Education, and Welfare Publication (NIH) No. 74-473, 1974.

Ullmann, K. "Leukoplakia Caused by Electrogalvanic Current Generated in Oral Cavity." *Ztschr. F. Stomatol.*, 30:802, 868 (1932).

Waerlauz, Z. "Tissue Reaction to Restorative Materials." *Oral Surgery, Oral Medicine and Oral Pathology*, 9:780-791 (1956).

Wakai, E. "Potential Difference Between Various Kinds of Metal Applied in Oral Cavity and Their Physiologic Effects." *Journal of the American Dental Association*, 23:1000 (June 1936).

West, E.S., and W.R. Todd. *Textbook of Biochemistry.* New York: The Macmillan Co., 1957.

White, A., P. Handler, E.L. Smith, and S. DeWitt. *Principles of Biochemistry.* New York: McGraw-Hill, 1959.

Wranglen, G., and J. Berendson. "Electrochemical Aspects of Corrosion Processes in the Oral Cavity with Special Reference to Amalgam Fillings." *Corrosion and Surface Protection of Metals.* Royal Institute of Technology, 1983.

# About the Author

Hal A. Huggins, D.D.S., M.S., received his dental degree from the University of Nebraska in 1962. There he met noted international lecturer Arne Lauritzen, L.D.S. Dr. Lauritzen asked Dr. Huggins to ghostwrite a book with him. The team spent the next five years researching an international textbook called Atlas of Occlusal Analysis, which was translated into five languages. The topic of the book is the original work on tempero mandibular joint (TMJ). Dr. Huggins was given the assignment of interviewing several of the noted dental and medical nutritionists of the day, and of writing the section on nutrition in dentistry.

Dr. Huggins became intrigued by blood chemistry and how it could be used to determine a patient's nutritional needs, as well as to monitor progress of a patient's treatment plan. He soon took blood chemistry interpretations into many aspects of dental degenerative disease, and he accidently found that all degenerative diseases had common denominators.

While expanding his chemistry interpretations, Dr.
Huggins met Olympio Pinto, C.D., of Rio de Janeiro, Brazil. Dr. Pinto introduced him to the concept of mercury
toxicity, and Dr. Huggins immediately found correlations
between dental materials and chemistry changes. His first
cases had "accidental" rapid improvements that captured
his attention and inspired him to delve into the depths of
chemistry, endocrinology, toxicology, and immunology to
develop what is now the most advanced technology for
treating dental material-stimulated degenerative and
autoimmune diseases.

Dr. Huggins entered into a Master of Science program
at the University of Colorado at Colorado Springs in 1985.
He graduated in 1989, and by that time had already incorporated many of the things he had learned into his private
practice. In 1990, he founded the Huggins Diagnostic Center, which embodies multiple health disciplines, including
medicine, dentistry, biochemistry, hematology, toxicology, pathology, nutrition, nursing, psychology, movement education, Feldenkrais (a gentle body discipline that
reintroduces the muscular system to the nervous system),
acupressure, massage, and sauna therapy, in one diagnostic and treatment facility, all under a team direction.

Dr. Huggins believes that mercury toxicity damages so
many areas that the team approach seems to be required
in order to cover the avenues found to stimulate recovery.
He hopes this will serve as a pattern for a future health-
care model.

Public interest in his techniques has brought him invi-
tations to speak in forty-six of the fifty United States and
thirteen foreign countries. Radio, television, and print
media have followed his research by requesting over 900
interviews in the past fifteen years.

# Index